So Old A Pain:
Depression in Fragments

Jerrad Peters

First published 2021
by Rowanvale Books Ltd
The Gate
Keppoch Street
Roath
Cardiff
CF24 3JW
www.rowanvalebooks.com

A CIP catalogue record for this book is available from the British Library.

Hardback ISBN: 978-1-913662-47-9

For JP

I will start at the end, as that's where it begins. And also because it doesn't matter, and it simply occurred to me to do so. If there's a better reason, I've yet to know of it. But one thing I've learned through all this is that it's never as it seems. That is, it's exactly what it seems and couldn't possibly be more precise. Only it's not. But it doesn't matter, I've already said that, I can say whatever I want. Come to think of it, we can go through it all in whatever order you choose. I couldn't care less. We can go from start to finish, which is really finish to start, only it isn't, or we can hopscotch like Cortázar[1], from this place to that, from here to there or there to here, and I'll even do one better: I won't tell you where to go next. There's always somewhere to go and someone telling you how to get there and I'm honestly quite tired of it all. Just tired, really. Come to think of it, we might as well go through it while you're sleeping. Yes, that would be best, I think. Because that's basically how I wrote it. Only it wasn't.

~ ~ ~

I have to go now. It's time.

Why do you have to go?

Because it's time.

Time for what?

Time to go.

But you just got here.

I know. But I have to go now. It's time.

How long will you be gone?

Could be months, maybe a year, maybe more. All I know is it's time.

Can I come with you?

No one can come where I'm going.

I could help you get there.

You couldn't.

I could help you get there and help you get back.

You couldn't. I have to go.

When will I see you again?

I don't know. It's time.

What should I tell them?

I'll explain it to them when they're older.

Please don't go.

I have to go. It's time. It's here.

You saw it coming?

Not until just now. It's time now.

I'm sorry.

Don't be sorry. I have to go.

I'm so sorry.

Please don't cry. It's time.

We'll wait for you.

I have to go now.

.

.

.

"It's the deep breath before the plunge."[2]

.

.

.

How did I get here?

.

.

.

"Sickness is the means by which an organism frees itself of foreign matter, so one must help it to be sick."[3]

~ ~ ~

How did I get here?

Does it matter? I don't owe you an explanation. How do any of us get anywhere? We are born, we do this and that, then we die. At one point or another, it doesn't matter which, we ask ourselves, "How did I get here?" At one point or another, it doesn't matter which, the question is put to us, "How did you get here?" It's the most human of questions, because it asks everything of us. And yet, it doesn't matter. I had little to do with it, you had little to do with it, we weren't consulted, though every now and then, at one point or another, it doesn't matter which, we tried to interject. But no one was listening, not then, not now, even if we planned our interjections, tried to anticipate the best moment to interrupt. It might have seemed a safe moment, or not, it doesn't really matter.

.

.

.

How did you get here?

Does it matter? You don't owe me an explanation, and I don't particularly care. You're here now, that's what matters. I asked you not to, but you came, you're here and I can't do anything about it, not now, it doesn't matter how you got here, you were doing this and that and now you're here, I wasn't consulted, you're here now. It tells me the story of your life, that you're here, with me, that we're together, making an interjection together, even if no one hears us, if no one is listening. I once heard it said that all things are plums and grief.

.

.

.

Are you comfortable? I'll just press play and we can get started.

.
.
.

What is going on here?

~ ~ ~

"I am my own parasite
I don't need a host to live
We feed off of each other
We can share our endorphins"[4]

.
.
.

Are you paying attention?

.
.
.

Do you understand?

~ ~ ~

I have thought a lot about how to bring you into it, how to introduce myself, to somehow let you know what's going on here. But that's the problem.

That's why we're doing this, I guess. To go through it all together, even though it's something that must be done alone. Not that there's anything unique in that, I guess, nothing special about it, we go through many things all by ourselves, most things, actually, very little about ourselves is known to others, we tell ourselves we wish to be known, to be understood and fully known, but if we had a choice we wouldn't change anything, not if it came right down to it. But we don't have a choice. Not even in the small things. We can taste the nectar of a plum and enjoy the pleasure of the flavour and texture and know that millions and tens and hundreds of millions of people have enjoyed similar pleasure since the very first plum tree sprouted from the ground and blossomed and bore fruit and was harvested. But only we have tasted what we are eating, no one else, not the particular piece of fruit and not with our particular taste buds, it's a solitary consumption and we don't think twice about it. Why would we? It's only eating. But what of bigger things? We certainly grieve alone. Others may grieve alongside, but it's only our bones that feel hollow, our guts that are twisted, our breath we can't catch, no one else's, not even a hug and the warmth of an embrace can thaw us, we mourn alone and we recover alone. We forget alone. And what we have forgotten is sealed inside the tomb we become.[5]

But that's the problem. There really is no point in saying anything. And if I had something to say, would you even care? We've only met. We don't know each other. We're strangers, you and I, and in that we're no different than anyone else in the history of the world. Besides, everything that has to be said has been said, what has to be written has been written, the librarians of Babel went insane and killed one another and themselves,[6] all things are plums and grief.

And so, we go ahead with it. I introduce myself to you and somehow let you know what's going on. You either listen or you don't, you pay attention or you don't, you understand or you don't, it's all the same to me. Because the solution to the problem, if we can call it that, is the same as it's always been, perhaps the one thing that has always been in common: there's nothing else to be done.

.

.

.

None of this is easy for me.

.

.

.

This is not a novel.

~ ~ ~

What is going on here?

.

.

.

I hate to break it to you, but I'm under no obligation to say. I don't have to tell you anything. Not about my present situation, not about my past, not about what I project for myself in the future, or where I project myself, my hopes and aspirations, if I have any of those, or my fears and anxieties, should I be afraid or uneasy, not any sense of foreboding about what is to come for me, assuming I have such a sense, not any interpretation of my life until this point and the situation I presently find myself in. I owe you none of that. You can draw your own conclusions based on what I tell you, but as to the little control I do, in fact, have I can exercise in the telling, I intend to take full advantage of that control. We are not on the same side.

I could tell you anything and you'd have to consider it. You wouldn't have to believe it, but you'd have to consider it, to at least incorporate it into the sum of what I'm telling you, to reserve some space for it in the process of drawing a conclusion, to assign it legitimacy, however perverse.

I am a walnut.

Am I not? I'm telling you that I am. And you've already furthered your consideration of me by the mere fact that I've told you that I am a walnut. You may not believe that I am a walnut, but the fact that I've told you that I am has influenced your consideration. Control. It's the little control I do, in fact, have. And you can't take it from me. No one can. It's the one thing no one can take.

.

.

.

What is going on here?

.
.
.

What is happening?

~ ~ ~

I just got up from my desk to check the brand of tea I'll be drinking. It's Uncle Lee's Organic Green Tea, UDSA-approved. I checked so I could tell you, and so I could distract myself a minute longer.

I just got up from my desk again because the kettle was boiling. The tea is steeping now, and I'm listening to Khachaturian's Piano Concerto in D-flat Major. I like how it begins. I'm back at my desk.

.

.

.

My tea is ready and I'm drinking it now.

.

.

.

I have finished my tea.

.

.

.

This is not a novel.

~ ~ ~

Last night I watched *Phantom Thread*. I wrote a poem about it that I will share with you now.

It is understated, except for the looking,
It is muffled piano,
It is patterned wallpaper,
It is important sounds.

It is lavish and sparse, quiet and clamorous,
It is asexual,
It is picking mushrooms,
You cook them in butter, but not too much.

It is a lantern in mist,
It is tree bark,
It is a gentle drunk,
It is a blush,
It is a scarf.

It is a defined chin,
The mushroom was poisonous,
It is melting butter,
The mushrooms are poisonous.

.
.
.

I have often thought it might be fun to write film reviews. I'm a huge Daniel Day Lewis fan.

.
.
.

What is happening?

~ ~ ~

Sometimes you talk to yourself. You just start talking, and it could be about anything, and it's a natural conversation about the outdoors or a passage from Vila-Matas or an encounter with someone. It's innocent enough to start, the conversation, and often quite persuasive and edifying and even lyrical. It's a mental underline of something you're thinking about, something important enough to merit a discussion, something you're trying to know better or avoid forgetting or bracing yourself for or against.

There's no harm in it, the conversation, at least there doesn't seem to be, but after a while, maybe a few days or a week or a month or two, the discourse has become one-sided and you can't get a word in edgewise, that is to say what you thought you might discuss with yourself is now being discussed without you, although it's you who is saying the words and thinking the thoughts that become the words, and you know things are not at all in a good way when you are speaking with someone and you think, after you have spoken with them, that "I didn't mean to say anything of the sort," or, "That isn't how I speak," or "I don't remember having such a voice," but it's out of your control to clarify because the other person is gone now and it was never really in your control, anyway.

The other person, perhaps having not seen you for a while, spoke briefly with you, who they know, at least as an acquaintance, but encountered a dialogue they were not prepared for, because they have never before encountered you on that plane of dialogue, and you are new to that plane of dialogue, yourself, although it is now the only dialogue and you don't need anyone else in order to have it, least of all that other person, just an acquaintance, and it's pretty much the narrative now, anyway.

So who cares. To hell with them. At no point was anyone else invited into the conversation, they approached you, and if you never see them again it won't be your fault. To hell with them. You were just out for a walk, getting some fresh air and having a talk, obeying some invisible pull, you have no control, it was never in your control, and to hell with everyone.

.

.

.

You need to pay attention.

.

.

.

Do you understand?

~ ~ ~

I have been looking at some old photographs. I keep them in a shoebox that I rarely take down from a shelf in my clothes closet, but earlier today I reached up to the shelf and took hold of the box and brought it down, heavy with photographs and forgotten things, a receipt, a folded, typewritten letter, a cork with a faded inscription or phrase in red ink, and carried it to my desk, where I opened it.

It's easy to forget the things we keep, what we save from certain times in our lives and don't throw away, whether we store them in a shoebox on a shelf or a dark corner of the basement or a disk that only an old computer can access. At one point we must have thought the things worth keeping, however ordinary. Perhaps we were tidying up and making room for the new, the useful, or maybe we were putting those things away, things that had once been immediate and meaningful but that eventually became antiques, tied to their times and a previous usefulness, although still alive with meaning.

Of course, what we knew when last we saw those things, whether in the shoebox or basement or on the computer screen before ejecting the disk, was that we were only about to store them, or hide them, to remove them from our attention with a promise to return to them, to the meaning they would maintain and nurture in the meantime. Because, we acknowledged, it wasn't us who assigned those things their meaning but rather those things that contained it and would continue to contain it so long as they existed in material form. It may have been that we

.

.

.

I had to stop there. I became quite melancholy writing those lines. I don't apologise. I owe you nothing.

.

.

.

I am lost. Not a word.[7]

.
.
.

This is not a novel.

~ ~ ~

"But that day I learned a skill at which I later excelled. I held back my despair..."[8]

~ ~ ~

"Do I contradict myself? Very well then, I contradict myself, I am large — I contain multitudes."

That's Lana Del Rey's Twitter bio. It's a quote of Walt Whitman's.

I like that.

.
.
.

You need to pay attention.

.
.
.

Do you understand?

~ ~ ~

I am inconsolably sad. Sad sad sad sad sad sad sad. Inconsolable inconsolable inconsolable inconsolable inconsolable inconsolable inconsolable. You need to understand what I'm telling you.

.

.

.

What am I?

Sad.

How am I?

Inconsolably sad.

.

.

.

You can't just move on. You can't read that and just move on. You might as well stop reading now. Whatever follows is right here in these lines. Whatever precedes them. You can't just read them and move on. You need to understand what I've told you, and, if you do read on, take them with you. Because there's nothing else you need to know. Nothing else I really need to tell you. Don't just gloss over it and keep on reading.

.

.

.

Sad.

Inconsolable.

You need to pay attention.

.

.

.

Inconsolably sad.

.

.

.

Do you understand?

.

.

.

Grief.

.

.

.

If I am grieving my own life, is there closure on the other side of that grief?

Closure for who?

.

.

.

I'm convinced most people are functionally illiterate.

~ ~ ~

"So how dark is it, really?"

Somebody asked me that the other day.

"So," given that I must ask, and that I assume I know what I'm asking and what I'm talking about, I might even have a shared experience, so I must understand.

"how dark," how removed from goodness and light and the daytime, if you don't mind me packing in all the tropes, but I've been there in the dark and emerged from it and into the light and the daytime, from where I'm asking you now, and from goodness, it's good to have this talk.

"is it," because it still is, it must be because I'm asking, I know what I'm asking and what I'm talking about, and it's in the present, it must be 'cause I'm asking, you're welcome.

"really?" For real, friend; as bad as all that, chum; a sticky wicket, guv'nor; buck up, old sport.

.

.

.

You need to understand what I'm telling you.

.

.

.

You need to pay attention.

~ ~ ~

"Look on the bright side is suicide
Lost eyesight I'm on your side
Angel left wing, right wing, broken wing
Lack of iron and/or sleeping"[9]

.

.

.

Thom Yorke said that "Kid A" was outside the fire and "Amnesiac" was inside the fire. I'm sure he said that, or something like that.

It's quiet inside the fire. Eerie. Even cool.

.

.

.

There is a place within me of which I know nothing. Now all things tend that way. I do not know what happens there.[10]

~ ~ ~

Burdens.

Burdensome things are hard to detach from. We adapt to our burdens and they become a part of our day-to-day. We might even love them. We love them even though they are bad for us.

They are burdensome.

.

.

.

It is good to live in pain.

.

.

.

I want to scream.

.

.

.

You need to understand what I'm telling you.

~ ~ ~

There comes a point when you realise that you have destroyed your life. The point where it's finally all peaceful and quiet and you have found closure. It's not the sort of closure which you intended from the start. It's not the closure got of ambition or endeavour. It's the place you land after you have slid so far down that you come to grips with the fact that it's futile to climb back up. It might be years before you reach that point. It is not easy to destroy a life.

.

.

.

If I were happy, what would I do about it? I would document it in one way or another. I would consider the cause of it and begin a volume about my happiness.

.

.

.

To self: Don't write it exactly from experience and keep a little room to manipulate it and make it at least a little less personal.

.

.

.

What is going on here?

.

.

.

I don't have to tell you anything.

~ ~ ~

There is a volume of memories that are getting worse and worse and becoming poison to me. I must write quickly before the whole volume is contaminated. There are memories that are worth saving but it will be difficult to coax them out without a lot of hurt.

.

.

.

Good memories to counteract. Good memories to take up space.

.

.

.

I am inconsolably sad.

~ ~ ~

You have always believed in me. You crave artistry and that wonderful river that brings it from the head to the hands. Those hands once folded and praying that it would all be revealed.

.

.

.

The great fight. The two great sides and the calm before the clash of forces.

.

.

.

Youth was the calm but we knew it all along, really. Now we have our armies against each other and all we can hope for is a victory one way or another. One of us will end and it and we will know who we really are.

You are the space and you are the world and this is the making of the history of you.

How you wish you would have made more of your immortality in youthful days. We might have tricked God and made a run with our immortality. We might have been gods ourselves in the world of men.

Now the armies are on the field and we get each other at least until the passage of this moment.

.

.

.

"I don't want to see you ever again."

.
.
.

I am inconsolably sad.

~ ~ ~

It is good to live in pain.

The world can produce only so much pain. Every person creates pain. They are bitter and selfish and they create pain by treating one another badly.

Many of them refuse their pain. They refuse to acknowledge that it exists and that it is theirs to bear. They are selfish and do not bear the pain that they create from their bitterness and they put it behind them and forgive themselves of their selfishness and eventually forget the pain they have created and are happy.

But it exists and it lingers and it must be bore.

Then those who are not as strong are saddened by the pain and pick it up and bear it. They bear it though it is not their own and theirs to carry. They cannot stand to see a world where pain goes unclaimed. So they claim it and bear it for those others and those others are happy because their pain is being carried and will never be on their shoulders.

But it is too much pain for the bearers to justify and they stumble under the weight of the pain and it is a bitter day each morning and their duties pale before the spectre of all the world's pain.

.

.

.

They are capable of so much good.

They were born capable of fashioning every good intention and fulfilling every good duty. It is not enough to bear that pain to which they have no responsibility. But they are incapacitated under its weight and bitterness and those futile attempts they make to be forgetful and happy and it ends in humiliation.

The humiliation is a consequence of the incapacity and they are vile and lazy and lacking and they carry the humiliation with the pain and none of it is theirs to bear but they are weak and romantic and the pain is colour to them. It is the colour the world creates and they are overcome by a craving for colour.

.

.

.

They crave colour and the artistry and that bitter river which brings it from the head to the hands.

.

.

.

The art of life is the art of avoiding pain.[11]

.

.

.

What is going on here?

.

.

.

You need to pay attention.

~ ~ ~

You are not awake to me anymore. You are only asleep. That is where I keep you and that is where you do not hurt me.

~ ~ ~

"I live in my suffering and that makes me happy. Anything that keeps me from living in my suffering is unbearable to me."[12]

.

.

.

This is not a novel.

~ ~ ~

I am looking at a photograph from 14 years ago. It shows three friends, seated on stools, and I'm in the middle. I hadn't seen this photograph until it was posted to Twitter last week. I waited until now to really examine it.

The two figures on either side of me are easily recognisable. They haven't changed much. No significant weight gain, or loss. Nothing about their clothing is peculiar. Neither is yet in their 40s, so they are still relatively young, as they were then. Their expressions are familiar, and both are looking at the camera, one turned slightly toward it and one facing it square on. But that's all I recognise. I know the setting, of course, but even it has changed somewhat. Still, I can feel the surface of the stools and even recall my friends' voices, even though I haven't spoken with them in quite some time. Voices, though, are recollections that come and go, recordings that are sometimes accurate when replayed and sometimes grainy, memories of memories, it's quite a random thing to remember voices when the voices you're trying to remember aren't speaking to you in the moment.

It's the middle figure I don't recognise. Me. Supposedly. Sure, I have changed physically, but we are always more critical of our own past appearances than we are of others', that's where our gaze centres — on ourselves — and we scrutinise what has changed and what hasn't, we wonder about our thoughts and our general situation in the moment the photograph was taken, we consider how much closer we are to death in the present, we either envy the younger person in the picture (for it is always a younger person) or despise them, we say things to ourselves like "if only I knew" or "if I could go back," it's an evocative exercise in looking.

The thing is, I'm completely unmoved by that middle figure. I know it's supposed to be me, but I can't comprehend him. My memory is comprehensive and precise, but I have no recollection of the seconds before the shutter closed and the seconds that followed. I don't remember being there. I must have erased it. Yet, there I sit, supposedly, looking somewhat downward, my lips turned slightly up, ever so slightly, in an expression that might otherwise be an impression of the Mona Lisa. I am thin, almost sickly thin, and the flash of the camera paints a glowing blotch on my pale forehead. Still, it's not the physique to which I'm apathetic, although I feel nothing when I survey it. No, my initial thought is, "That person never existed." Of course, he obviously did exist, for there he sits, but I cannot extrapolate him, I cannot bring him into the future, nor can I follow him into the past. It's as if he was only ever there, neither born nor hurtling towards death. The picture was taken and there he was.

So who am I, then? If that's not me, then where was I, what was I, 14 years ago when those three figures sat next to one another and posed for a photograph? Did I only begin sometime after that? And what of before? If that is, indeed, me, then a chunk of me is missing, a section of my time in the world simply isn't, the me that I call myself, to which I identify, began sometime after that, but not long after, maybe a few months based on the date of the photograph, and then things become quite apparent, and then I forget nothing. Except what I choose to forget. I can visualise a rubber eraser, and when I choose to forget something I rub it away with the eraser and blow away the bits of rubber, and then it is no more. I lay out the text of the thing I want to forget and take my eraser to it. Perhaps that's what I did with the time of the photograph.

.

.

.

"...three friends..."

~ ~ ~

The most heartbreaking thing in life is watching a child become self-aware. From that point onward they are hurtling toward death. I can't imagine a more tragic thing.

.

.

.

I am inconsolably sad.

~ ~ ~

Keep me far away
Hold me far away from you
Say it's all nostalgia
The unfortunate side of you

~ ~ ~

I have the Vatican's Click to Pray app on my mobile. The current prayer intention of Pope Francis is "that Christians, followers of other religions, and all people of goodwill may promote peace and justice in the world."

"Click To Pray."

"Thank You For Praying."

.

.

.

"...all people of goodwill..."

.

.

.

We all at some time grow unutterably weary of being who we are and who we were.[13]

~ ~ ~

One day my head did not feel right. It felt like something was opening up my head and pouring a chemical into it. I could feel it pouring in and then I could feel nothing but it pour in, slowly and thick-pouring, crying and the sad, desperate pouring. It would pour in and then when my head was full of it, it would go down into my chest. Then it would be hard to breathe and then my stomach would hurt. Then it would go down to my feet and hollow out my legs on the way down, and my arms, too, like chicken bones, and without skin, skeletal. I would lie there in the cold, sweating some of the chemical from my body, sweating there in the freezing cold and more and more chemical pouring in and spreading from my head to my chest to my stomach to my limbs and more and more of it no matter how much of it I sweat.

At first I thought the chemical was a person. It was a person opening up my head and pouring themselves into my head and down and through my body. They were a person because they had feelings and talked and took up space in my head and in my body that they wouldn't let me have. They had thoughts and feelings and they said things out of my mouth. Sometimes they hurt people with the things they said. They had thoughts and feelings and they always wanted to be alone with their thoughts. They thought about terrible things and the things they thought about made me very sad. They had feelings that I had never felt and that I couldn't understand, feelings that didn't have words to be described by, feelings that kept pouring into my head and down through my body, taking up the space they wouldn't let me have, that space in my own head and my own body that was kept from me, locked and heavy with chemicals and feelings. The space would fill up and the thought-chemical would pour into my lungs and stomach, sweating and hard breathing and not eating, and down through my body and into my limbs, aching limbs and hollow bones and immobilised and not moving.

Sometimes it would stop pouring itself in. It would all stop and it would leave me tired and afraid, tired from fighting off the chemical and sweating and being the body for a treacherous thought-chemical and carrying around a space for it in my head and in my body. I would be tired and afraid of it pouring in again. I would know that it might come and I was very afraid, afraid of having horrible thoughts and tight breathing and not eating and not moving, afraid that I was slowly losing my head and my body to the pouring-in chemical.

I was afraid all the time and I waited in fear for it to start pouring in again. Sometimes I hoped it would start to pour in so that I would not have to be afraid. Then it started to pour in and I hoped I would die so that I'd never have the horrible thoughts or struggle to breathe or be sick through my body or afraid. Then some of me did die. Some of me was erased, blotted out from history, rubbed out by a rubber eraser, the bits of rubber blown away and scattered by the wind to nowhere and nothing, life degree zero, the dead part, the erased part, the missing part, the void, the void of the deep, the colour of desolation, the pit in between, a howl from the pit, a trauma, a trauma, a sealed tomb with the devil watching over, the devil sitting on the seal of the tomb, a hell, a trauma, abyss, a trauma.

.

.

.

"I will give you life."

.

.

.

"The World is a closed thing, cyclical, resonant, eternally-returning."[14]

.

.

.

I don't owe an explanation.

~ ~ ~

I WANT TO SCREAM.

~ ~ ~

I have no future.

~ ~ ~

I should kill myself tonight.

~ ~ ~

I don't owe an explanation and I won't bear the balance of guilt.

~ ~ ~

"I am depressed by the sight of furrows — including those made by my pen. The recurrence of the seasons and of their effects illustrates the stupidity of nature and of life, which can persist only by repeating itself. I think, too, of the monotonous efforts required to trace lines in the heavy soil, and I am not surprised that the obligation inflicted on man of 'earning his bread by the sweat of his brow' should be considered a harsh and degrading punishment."[15]

.

.

.

"I am depressed by the sight of furrows — including those made by my pen."

.

.

.

What is the point of these lines, these pages I am making for you, that you are reading? I hope, to borrow from Roland Barthes, and to perhaps do so audaciously (as if there was another way to borrow from Barthes), that this text desires you. But how are you going about your reading? Are you paying attention? Do you understand?

.

.

.

"I know these are only words, but all the same..."[16] (italics Barthes')

.

.

.

"I hope..."

An odd pairing of words. Can it be that my remaining expectation of life is that you will read these pages?

.

.

.

Are you paying attention?

.

.

.

Do you understand?

~ ~ ~

There is nothing outside my apartment that interests me. Inside I have my books, my tea, my music. There is nothing outside I want to do.

~ ~ ~

I am reading Kate Briggs' essay, *This Little Art*. I am drinking tea and listening to Billy Taylor. Briggs returns often in her writing to Robinson Crusoe's construction of a table. She is using the table, she says, as "a device to think with".

Are these lines, these pages, a device? Only, perhaps, if you take them as a whole and use them as a lens, a lens through which to see the world, my world, to interpret it. You can maybe use the lens and look through it and try to place yourself somewhere in the world in which I live.

I'd like you to do that.

~ ~ ~

I'd like to return to the world of the living.

"I'd," I still have a sense of myself.

"like," there is still enjoyment, or at least the ability to imagine enjoyment, to remember it.

"to return," I was once there, and I can remember being there.

"to the world," it is a place "to" which I must go, because I am not currently there, it is a world, an experience of being, and I've been there before.

"of the living," I've been there before, in that living world, that lived experience of being, but where I am now is not that world, it is the world of the dead.

If I am in the "world" of the dead, I must also be in mourning. I am grieving.

~ ~ ~

Briggs writes a lot about Robinson Crusoe's table. It makes me think of Heidegger. My thoughts go to Heidegger because I have a recollection of him using a table as a device through which to discuss art. Only, as I reach for the Heidegger on my shelf, it is a temple that he uses as the device and not a table.[17] Why did I think it was a table he used? Perhaps I reduced the temple to a table so as to make his illustration smaller in scale, more in front of me.

Art, he writes, "is the becoming and happening of truth."

And he writes about Van Gogh's shoes,[18] the true shoes. I'll try to think of shoes the next time Briggs talks about Robinson Crusoe's table.

Heidegger might say these lines, these pages, are truer than my condition. That gives me comfort.

.
.
.

What is going on here?

~ ~ ~

I had a dream last night that scared me. I don't remember the dream, only colours of it—reds, blacks, whites, in flashes. I remember that it scared me. I have been scared all day.

.
.
.

"I don't want to see you ever again."

~ ~ ~

On the very next page of *This Little Art*, Briggs cites a passage by Jacques Derrida that references some uses of the table in philosophy: "from Plato to Heidegger, from Kant to Ponge, and so many others."

So I wasn't wrong about Heidegger's table. I just couldn't find it. Maybe I'm not going totally crazy.

.

.

.

I nearly spelled "Kant" "Kante". This afternoon I watched Chelsea-Arsenal, and N'Golo Kante slipped on the pitch and allowed Gabriel Martinelli to break forward and score.

.

.

.

I couldn't use my computer for several hours late this morning and early this afternoon and watched the first half of the match on my phone. My laptop is old and can't hold a charge. It overheats at the slightest bit of work. And the modem is struggling to pick up the wireless signal.

.

.

.

Nothing works for me.

~ ~ ~

I am looking into a world unborn and formless, that needs to be ordered and shaped.[19]

But I can't shape it, even though I have a sense of what the shape should be. And I can't order it, even if I once functioned within that order.

The world I inhabit doesn't exist.

I am, as Michel Foucault writes in *Madness and Civilization*, "confronting a world recognized as such by implicit reference to a reality that has become inaccessible".

If I can't access that reality, do I exist? Did I?

~ ~ ~

There's no tea in my cupboard and I'm not sure what to do. I don't want to go to the store. I don't want to go anywhere. But I'm irritated. I'm irritated because I want a cup of tea and can't have one. And I'm confused. I'm confused about running out of tea and confused, confused. My arms feel funny. I've become quite weak.

.

.

.

I am the Minister of Information. You know only what I want you to know.

.

.

.

Are you paying attention? Do you understand?

~ ~ ~

It has been 13 years since my first treatments.

.

.

.

One of Ludwig Binswanger's patients, writes Foucault[20], "was caught between the wish to fly, to float in an ethereal jubilation, and the fear of being trapped in a muddy earth that oppressed and paralyzed her...the world had become 'silent, icy, dead'...It was this that provided the background of the psychosis and of the symptoms (fear of getting fat, anorexia, affective indifference) that led her over a morbid period of thirteen years to suicide."

.

.

.

"...silent, icy, dead..."

.

.

.

Thirteen years.

.

.

.

Am I at the end of the same morbid period?

~ ~ ~

Carl Ludwig Nietzsche died when he was 36. His son, Friedrich, recalled him as "delicate, lovable and morbid, like a being destined to pay this world only a passing visit."[21] Friedrich's health also declined at the same point of adulthood: "…in the 36th year of my life I arrived at the lowest point of my vitality—I still lived, but without being able to see three paces in front of me." He quit his job and "lived through the summer like a shadow" and "*as* a shadow" during the winter (italics Nietzsche's).

.

.

.

I am 36. I quit my job and lived through the summer like a shadow and *as* a shadow during the winter. Am I, like Carl Ludwig, destined to pay this world only a passing visit?

.

.

.

I am at the lowest point of my vitality.

.

.

.

The world is loud, like the periphery of a great fire, but in the middle of the fire, where I am, it is quiet, even cool.

.

.

.

Nietzsche said silence is bad for the stomach.

~ ~ ~

"I won my own pet virus
I get to pet and name her
Her milk is my shit
My shit is her milk"[22]

~ ~ ~

I am selfish.

I want to be happy and so much so that I am obsessed with happiness.

I am always alert for it.

I go to bed and expect to find it in the morning; when I don't, I expect to find it before the next morning.

I will do anything for it.

I will do anything if there is even a chance that doing it will bring happiness.

I am always alert for it and always think that I am one decision away from it.

I am selfish and greedy about my happiness.

I will do anything to have it.

.
.
.

"And sometimes I think I kill relationships for art
I start up all this shit to watch 'em fall apart
I pay my bills with it, I watch 'em fall apart
Then pay the price for it, I watch 'em fall apart, but

Oh, I just wanna be fucking happy, oh, oh, oh
Oh, I just wanna be fucking happy, yeah"[23]

~ ~ ~

"You know perfectly well that Guy always wanted to be unhappy."[24]

What was it about Guy? Why was it assumed to be known "perfectly well" that he "always wanted to be unhappy"?

Why "always"?

Perhaps, ever since he had been "known", he had tended toward melancholy. Maybe that was a sort of natural disposition for Guy. Perhaps he didn't smile much. I've known several people like that, although I wouldn't say that they'd "always wanted to be unhappy".

What if he was a failed artist of some kind, or even a working and successful artist? Many artists have been described as "unhappy", and certainly melancholy. There has always been something a bit off with the good ones. We make art, explains Umberto Eco in his lecture "On Some Forms of Imperfection in Art", delivered at La Milanesiana in 2012, because we are imperfect. I wonder if Guy, knowing he was imperfect and really, truly knowing, and knowing as knowing a great secret, such as the secret that he would one day die, a secret very few really, truly know, found the burden of his imperfection and his secret too great a burden to bear, and was unhappy as a result. And he would, in that case, have wanted to be unhappy, because there would have been no other way for him to be. And the art that he made — there is no reference to his being an artist, although if he really, truly bore the secret of his imperfection, he would have kept his art a secret, a paradox — would, if its existence wasn't a secret and he happened to show it in a gallery for example, convey profound unhappiness. "Here is an artist who is unhappy," the viewers and critics might have said. "He has always been that way and has wanted to be so. It's who Guy *is*."

Of course, Guy might also have been the type of fellow who simply wore the air of unhappiness as a sort of accessory, the way one might wear a hat or a scarf. In this instance, "You know perfectly well that Guy always wanted to be unhappy" would tend to be an insult, or at least a light-hearted descriptor.

Then again, the speaker is claiming that "You know perfectly well", so it must have been a sincere unhappiness. I'll at least give Guy the benefit of the doubt on that score. In any event, I feel badly for Guy. I'd like to know more about him, to pursue him.

I don't think anyone pursued Guy. I find that heartbreaking.

~ ~ ~

I haven't eaten a vegetable in weeks. This is also a physical decline. I am very weak. When this is over I'm going to have to learn to walk again.

.

.

.

How do I tell them how my body feels?

The heaviness just inside both of my shoulders? The tautness of the underside of my forearms? The pain all through my legs? The aching of my upper jaw towards my cheeks? The fear in my lungs—I can't think of another word for it; maybe a sort of "gnawing" from within them to the outside, outside my chest? The felt barricade of my skull, like a kind of wall or sturdy panelling, unbreakable to any good thought that might relieve the agony of the rest of me? A brain that bruises at the slightest memory?

Do I have to tell them?

.

.

.

"When this is over..."

~ ~ ~

I was watching the series *Thieves of the Wood*, or *De Bende van Jan de Lichte* in its original Dutch. There was to be a hanging, and they paraded the convicted—each of them innocent—through the main square of Aalst to the scaffold. I couldn't wait to see them hung. I wanted to see how they awaited their deaths on the gallows and how quickly they died once the hangman pulled the lever. Would they struggle and writhe in the noose? Would there be snapping sounds of their necks being broken? Would they defecate? Christopher Heyerdal urinated as his character was hung in *Hell on Wheels*. But his character was guilty. These were innocent.

.

.

.

"With failing eyes K. could still see the two of them immediately before him, cheek leaning against cheek, watching the final act. 'Like a dog!' he said; it was as if the shame of it must outlive him."[25]

.

.

.

I've been to Kafka's little house in the Golden Lane at Prague Castle.

.

.

.

"The grim
egoism (egotism)
of mourning
of suffering"[26]

~ ~ ~

There are a lot of expressions about "living in the past", and most of them are quite awful, the sort of fluff you'll see on Pinterest or read in the memoirs of people who didn't, or don't, think much about anything at all, let alone "time".

"You can't live in the past. There's nothing you can do about," is a particularly bad one, courtesy of the former tennis star Martina Navratilova. But it's not nearly as bad as this travesty, courtesy of the American newspaper columnist and playwright George Ade: "Nothing is improbable until it moves into past tense." What does that even mean? Johnny Cash, who I have a lot of time for, offered this unfortunate attempt at wisdom: "Close the door on the past." For what it's worth, I don't think he believed a word of what he was saying.

Obviously, none of us can "live" in the past. The very notion is a contrariety. But we all of us live "on" the past. Memories are the DNA of time.

Is it so far-fetched to believe that a scientist or researcher of this particular DNA would be unhappy, would be inconsolably sad?

I wonder if Guy wasn't a scientist or researcher of memory DNA.

Personally, I like this quote of Stephen Hawking's: "The past, like the future, is indefinite and exists only as a spectrum of possibilities."

Nailed it on the head, our Stephen.

.

.

.

Are you paying attention?

~ ~ ~

There's a scene in *Vivir sin Permiso*[27] that I really like. José Coronado's character, Nemo, is looking out the window of his house. He has recently learned that he has Alzheimer's, and he's thoughtfully looking out the window when his wife, Chon, sees him from the hallway and gazes at the back of him, watching him watch whatever he's watching. Perhaps he's thinking of her, she must wonder, or their children, or the family business Nemo is trying to straighten out before he's incapacitated. But he's thinking none of that. He's not looking aimlessly out the window but at a boat in the yard, a boat he used to row with his young love, the love of his life whom he left to pursue the monied Chon, the recently deceased Ada, with whom he had a daughter. Chon is looking at Nemo who is looking at Ada and their daughter, at the boat, a straightforward metaphorical vessel. Pun intended.

But no one is looking back. Ada is not looking back at Nemo; Nemo is not looking back at Chon. They're both of them looking at death.

("Yes, but there is also life. There is the daughter, Lara." That's what I want you to tell me.)

.

.

.

We do very peculiar things while we're alive. No one sees us do them. No one sees where we are looking.

~ ~ ~

There is no interaction that isn't ultimately a wound, and nothing reopens those wounds, rips off the scabs, quite like photographs, especially old photographs.

.

.

.

I have been looking at old photographs. Some are of me; some are of other people; some are of me with other people. "They have their whole lives before them; but also they are dead [today], they are then already dead [yesterday]. At the limit, there is no need to represent a body in order for me to experience this vertigo of time defeated."[28] "In the sentence, 'She's no longer suffering,' to what, to whom, does that 'she' refer? What does that present tense mean?"[29] "Now I claim to know — and to be able to say adequately — why, in what she consists. I want to outline the loved face by thought, to make it into the unique field of intense observation; I want to enlarge this face in order to see it better, to understand it better, to know its truth (and sometimes, naively), I confide this task to a laboratory."[30]

.

.

.

"To what, to whom, does that 'she' refer?"

.

.

.

I once threw out a diary of mine. It contained the best material I have ever written, but of course I can say that now it's burned, or decomposing, or lingering in a landfill. I sometimes wish I hadn't thrown it out, and a part of me still searches for it. But I know why I threw it out and I knew then. It was prophecy, an oracle of the damned. I threw it out to prevent hurt, to somehow avoid the wound, to escape what was inevitable. There is no interaction that isn't ultimately a wound; there is no polishing the scratches that tell us how we feel.

.

.

.

"There's so many things I want to share with you
So much is there to make me miss you"[31]

~ ~ ~

It is a much better view in the summer.

The worst part of the winter view was longing for this one.

It's not even a view so much as an experience. Tomorrow seems so far away when you see the night like this.

Far away like you're looking for it and can't see it for the darkness.

(Starlight flashing off the crystal and tabletop and in each other's eyes and flickering off the river like raindrops hitting the ground under a streetlight in a Childe Hassam painting, old trees thick and dark in the night, dipping leaves into the river and stirring the starlight.)

We always analyse everything so particularly.

We have our own way of understanding each other and making something out of anything.

It's like our own little civilisation.

I would say we are quite civilised.

Civilised for the purpose of being amusing to ourselves and playing with what we really think the other is secretly thinking.

There are no secrets. We're just holding on to these last moments.

Our history is an aggregate of last moments.[32]

Do they have to be the last ones? Can't we just sit here a while longer?

Let's risk it. Let's pretend the day will never come.

It will be like a dream.

Like a dream we tell to each other, a secret code.

And when we tell it we will always be here.

Such a precious dream, like a scripture.

A dream is a scripture, and many scriptures are nothing but dreams.[33]

I want to keep dreaming.

If only we could.

It's not that easy, is it.

It's not.

Then let's go. Let's not prolong it.

You can go. I'd like to stay here a while yet.

You can stay.

Will you come back?

I have some things to do first.

I'll wait for you here.

Right here?

Right here.

~ ~ ~

Good memories to counteract.

Good memories to take up space.

~ ~ ~

If I were to die, I'd want my body to be placed in Nemo's boat, floating by myself, come what may.

.

.

.

"If I were to die…"

.

.

.

To what, to whom, does that "I" refer?

.

.

.

"…my body…"

.

.

.

Whose body? What does that even mean? It can't be mine if I am dead. The body that used to be mine? The body that my "I" used to inhabit? But who is talking?

.

.

.

What is going on here?

~ ~ ~

I bought a new laptop the other day. It was nice to leave my apartment and go to the store and buy a laptop like a regular person. I still have my old laptop, as well as my very first laptop. There were two others as well, but one stopped working and the other I gave away. I'll keep my old laptop and my very first laptop until I'm unable to use them. I don't like throwing things out. I have so few things.

.

.

.

I'm tired of cooking, tired of using the toilet, tired of thinking. It takes me two days to generate the energy to do my laundry. My clothes are soiled. I am disgusting, a disgusting creature, mud is my home. You can't see me. I'm lying in mud and mud is my home.

.

.

.

Do you understand what I'm telling you?

.

.

.

You need to pay attention.

.

.

.

"I am my own parasite."

~ ~ ~

In conversation with a friend: "So what? Jerrad Peters went and offed himself. Would I be surprised? No. And you know what? You won't. You would have already. And if you do, would I be surprised? No. Would I be upset? Sure. But I wouldn't be surprised. Went and offed himself, did JP? Well, you would have already."

I hugged him.

.

.

.

"...with a friend."

.

.

.

"If you're gonna kill yourself,
Then to save face get on with it."[34]

.

.

.

"I live in my suffering and that makes me happy."

.

.

.

Are you paying attention?

.

.

.

Do you understand?

~ ~ ~

"You have seen things and known things that are not meant to be seen and known and felt things that have no words to describe the feelings. But I am proud of you. This is a happy story. It is a special thing. You are describing to me and to all of the people and you must never stop describing it and telling us about it. Because we have never been there. We don't want to go there and we are terrified of it and we are afraid of the people who have been there and seen it and understood it and felt it. So come back to us and tell us about it. Come back to us. And if you can't, yell it from where you are. But please come back to us. It's time to come back to us."

.

.

.

That's what I want you to say, to tell me. If you could say it right here, right now, and really, truly mean it, then none of this would be necessary.

.

.

.

It would still be necessary. I live in my suffering and that makes me happy. You can't see me. I'm lying in mud, and mud is my home.

~ ~ ~

You have something I do not have.

.

.

.

I want to interrupt you when you're having dinner with your family after a long day. I want to barge right in and upset the table, toss it right over and send food flying everywhere. On your face and your children's faces. And then I want to grab you by the hair and pull you up and slap you in the face. I want to pin you down to the table and stuff food inside your mouth and spit in your mouth. I want to take your steak knife and thrust it into your leg and scratch your face. Maybe you'll die. Maybe you won't. It's all the same to me.

.

.

.

There is no interaction that isn't ultimately a wound.

~ ~ ~

There are moments when you wake up and you feel no different than when you went to sleep. You went to bed heavy and burdened by something heavy in the head and you wake up and the heavy thing is still there. You might have had a few too many the night before, which didn't help; but it's not that morning-after-a-few-too-many kind of heaviness. It's a heaviness that pins you to the bed and you are too heavy to get out of bed and get into the day.

You feel that the bright day demands too much of you and your head is too burdened by heaviness to get out of bed and pull apart the bright, sun-shining-through-the-window drapes. You lie in bed and worry about how to get rid of the heaviness; how to feel the warmth of the sun on your face; how to move from your bed to the window to washing up at the sink and shaving and putting on clothes. And so you run through the things you have to do during the day. All the things that keep you from the next going-to-bed and being pinned in the safe bed.

You run it all through, a trial run, a trial, and maybe it won't be heavy anymore. You run through every detail and every future motion to see if there's anything to be afraid of. Sometimes you become a little less heavy and a little less afraid. Sometimes you don't. And then, even though it's the morning and you're awake, it's really not and you really aren't. Will today be the day, you wonder. Will it be today. And then you clean the apartment because you don't want them to find it messy if it is.

.

.

.

"Help me make it through the night,
I don't care who's right or wrong.
I don't try to understand,
Let the devil take tomorrow,
Lord tonight I need a friend."[35]

~ ~ ~

Claudia Traisac, who plays Lara Balarés in *Vivir sin Permiso*, posted the song "Run from Me" by Timber Timbre to her Instagram account.

"Run from me, darlin',
Run, my good wife.
Run from me, darlin',
You better run for your life."

~ ~ ~

Think of it like a strong wind—*galinn* in Old Norse[36], "mad"," "insane", gale force but stronger. You are on a cliff's edge and endeavouring to walk forward to surer ground, but you are struggling against the wind, the wind that brings mist and droplets of rain that blow into your eyes. You stoop to take each step more sturdily, but the wind keeps getting stronger and through the mist and rain, now more than droplets, you can barely see in front of you. You pull your coat more tightly around you so as to keep dry, but in doing so you lose your balance, your carefully calculated balance and planned advance of steps, and you fall backward off the cliff. And as you look up from whence you've fallen, the last thing you see is the edge of the cliff. It's the last thing you see, your final memory of a memory, and it's all there ever was.

~ ~ ~

How do I tell them how my body feels?

The twisting in my gut from being folded up for days, weeks, months at a time. The stiffness in my neck that pulls down a line to my shoulder, also stiff and hurting. The overwhelming, devastating fatigue. So much of this is physical.

Do I have to tell them?

.

.

.

"Yesterday is dead and gone,
And tomorrow's out of sight,
And it's sad to be alone."[37]

~ ~ ~

I know this is a short book. I'm self-conscious about it. It would have been better to write a longer book.

"Well I DO say, LOOK at this VERY LONG BOOK! Just LOOK at it! It MUST be IMPRESSIVE! It must WEIGH as much as SARTRE and can WEIGH your GROCERIES![38]

But it took more than a year to write. And in real time, too. More than 13 years, actually. Back to the first time. The first real time. Written by hand on the 26th floor and some of it before that, in the secret time.

It's a volume. Take your time with it. Try to understand.

.
.
.

Are you paying attention?

~ ~ ~

"Run from me, darlin',
You better run for your life.
Run, run, run, run, run,
Run, run, run, run, run,
Run, run, run, run, run,
Run, run, run, run, run."[39]

~ ~ ~

As I write this, I am listening to an hour-long recording that supposedly captures the street sounds of Rome. Yes, it's super lame, and no, I don't care. I'm obsessed with Rome, and I think I'm obsessed with it because it's the last place I was before it all went to pieces. If we were sitting across from one another, I'd tell you, in words you can understand, that it's "the last place I was happy". More accurately, it's the last "time" I was "happy", and I suppose I just happened to be in Rome then. That was 18 months ago. It seems longer — only, it doesn't.

The thing is, I can recall my life of 18 months ago more clearly than my life of eight months ago, or even four months ago. I can recall walking upstairs after breakfast and opening the tall shutters and hanging my laundry out the window to dry. And then going back down to the street and having a cappuccino and smoking a cigarette. I can remember exact trees in exact places and where the streets incline and where they slope. Then, on a Friday before dawn, I left Rome and the streets and returned home and to it all going to pieces. It still took a few more months to fall apart, but at the point in my memory where there starts to be only mist, I know it was under way.

One morning I was having my cappuccino in Piazza Navona, there is nothing quite like the Roman blue of the morning, and the next evening I went to sleep in my own bed. I didn't know it yet, although when I look back to that time I can almost visualise the mist descending, a chemical mist, thickening quickly and then enveloping everything, when I look back I can see only the mist, toxic and thick, and I can't see myself through it, though I must have been there, trying to see out, and it continued to thicken, and when I look back I can't locate my position, the compass would have spun confusedly, as if I had arrived at some signal zero, the fixed point, original, because that's when, in looking back, all directions, ups and downs, morality, the density of presence, amalgamated at the fixed point, undifferentiated, only the fixed point and the mist.

That's what I see when I try to look back to that time, but my gaze is distorted, warped, a memory of a memory, familiar yes, familiar in its agony, forgive me for trying to look around it, to watch myself opening the tall shutters and hanging my laundry out the window to dry. It's just easier that way.

.

.

.

"I measure every Grief I meet
With narrow, probing eyes —
I wonder if It weighs like Mine —
Or has an easier size.

"I wonder if They bore it long —
Or did it just begin —
I could not tell the Date of Mine —
It feels so old a pain — [40]

.

.

.

"...so old a pain..."

~ ~ ~

Nietzsche was right about the stomach, by the way.

~ ~ ~

"Look on the bright side is suicide
Lost eyesight I'm on your side
Angel left wing, right wing, broken wing
Lack of iron and/or sleeping"[41]

.
.
.

I know that this will one day kill me.

~ ~ ~

At the bottom of a small, wooden box in which I keep bank notes and coins from Asia, Central America and pre-Eurozone Europe, I found a poem. It was at the very bottom of the box, where it must have looked up at the face of His Excellency Count Ioannis Antonios Kapodistrias[42] for 16 years or more before I found it. At least, that's about how old I date it. The neat, intentional handwriting suggests it was first scribbled on a piece of notepaper, likely at a café, before being copied and arranged into three stanzas, the first two with numbered lines, 10-9-9-8-10, the syllables of each line.

It's a poem that I wrote when I wrote a lot of poems, that anxious activity of youth, many of them awful and embarrassing, not only the poems themselves, but also the thoughts that brought them to the page. This one isn't any better than the rest, although I must have valued it and the thoughts that brought it to the page, I saved it after all, preserving it on top of coins from China, Thailand, Mexico, Dominican Republic, Italy, Greece, Great Britain, The Netherlands and Turkey, and beneath notes from the same places, as well as Burma (now Myanmar) and Hong Kong, the bottom note worth 500 drachmas. The handwriting is neat, but the lines filled with nonsense to achieve the syllabic goal, I was obsessed with syllables. Still, there are two lines that give me goosebumps, not because the lines have any literary value, but because they seem to foretell something, they are prophecy.

"It's fit that my reward should be disguised
Appear to only eyes whose gaze may pierce the past"

I have departed from the 10-9-9-8-10, and indeed there is a stroke through one of the nines. My "reward" is clearly "happiness", or at least tolerable living, I was absolutely miserable when I wrote the poem, a wreck, and my state would worsen over two more years, careening towards a nervous breakdown, just before which it could have gone either way. "Disguised" I think is what I would now call "distorted", a peering into a thickening mist, memories of memories, unattainable. I can't see it, I admit as much in the next line, "only eyes" are clearly not "my eyes", although I wish they were, and perhaps I still hope, at the time of writing, that my vision will improve or the mist, the disguise, will disintegrate. "Pierce the past", well, that's my obsession, isn't it, as if in the past I'll find the hidden thing, the "reward", perhaps in that primordial soup, the original pool, the embryonic liquid that we, like fish, flopping on the shore, awkwardly and pathetically twitch toward, our lives depending on it. The thing is, I wasn't thinking these thoughts back then, about 16 years ago, it was simply an anxious poem, it just came out, likely on a piece of notepaper at a café, later copied, a prophecy, although not a self-fulfilling one, I must have quickly placed the page at the bottom of the box, I only found it now because I was looking for something else.

The text is rich with meaning, even if the writing of it wasn't. But then, that's true of many texts. What I find eerie about this one is that, encode-decode, I've composed an open text to myself, a text that was meant to be found, but not until now.

.
.
.

Are you paying attention?

.
.
.

Do you understand?

~ ~ ~

Bob Dylan released a new song today: "I Contain Multitudes."

"Got a tell-tale heart like Mr. Poe
Got skeletons in the walls of people you know
I'll drink to the truth and the things we said
I'll drink to the man that shares your bed
I paint landscapes, and I paint nudes
I contain multitudes."[43]

~ ~ ~

The world has coronavirus[44] and has slowed to my speed. I am selfish and enjoying the world around me, the slow world, the sick world, the dying world. People are sick, and I am enjoying that. People are dying, and I am enjoying that, too. The world is a contagion, and I am my own parasite. I am disgusting, a disgusting creature, mud is my home.

~ ~ ~

A text just I sent to a friend: "I am having a cappuccino and the café is spinning 'Hey Ya'."[45] I have ventured out into the city and am reading at a café and having a cappuccino at a café for the first time in many months. They will close the cafés soon, but I was here. Let the record show. Quite suddenly, as if overnight, the world has opened up to me, the sick, welcoming world, and I am out and about in it as one healthy, as one who knows his way around the world.

.

.

.

"…to a friend…"

~ ~ ~

The pandemic has given me wind. For the first time in 11 months I rode a bus, went downtown and sat in a café with a cappuccino. The Italians are quarantined[46] and cannot get their cappuccinos. The best cappuccino I ever had was in Rome. I was staying on Via Angelo Poliziano on the Esquiline Hill, a short walk to both Parco del Colle Oppio and Basilica di Santa Maria Maggiore, which is at the Esquiline summit and where a sacred relic of the Holy Crib is kept in a reliquary. I have a print of *Salus Populi Romani*[47] and a rosary from the Basilica.

.

.

.

Italy is my favourite country in the world. When this is over I want to go to Milan.

.

.

.

"When this is over…"

~ ~ ~

March 19, 2020

Dear Diary,

Today I wrote a newspaper column about the resumption of sport, and what it will look like, once the world has either gone back to normal or commenced a new, post-coronavirus normal. I wrote it in one sitting and weaved in some passages of Balzac that speak to our ability to accept change, to be adaptable, to quickly fill voids, to move on.

I haven't felt so clear-headed in almost a year.

COVID-19 has given me wind.

.
.
.

I don't owe you an explanation.

~ ~ ~

The world is still. It is moving at my speed and I feel at home in it.

I look out my window, and there is no one. I go for a walk, and there is no one. The canals in Venice are clean and the Shanghai sky is clear. There is a bright sun and a new season. There are birds. I am watching a lot of BBC Earth. There is panic on the news channels but the world is still and I wouldn't change anything. Not a single thing. Not the panic, not the fear, not the grief, not the despair. None of it is mine. It's your turn now, and I enjoy seeing you like this. I wouldn't change that, either. It's your turn now. We're opposites, you and I, and when you panic, fear, grieve and despair, I am still. Still and Venice and sun and BBC Earth.

.

.

.

My

speed.

~ ~ ~

Social distancing.[48]

What does Social Distancing mean?[49]
This means making changes in your everyday routines in order to minimize close contact with others, including:
- avoiding crowded places and non-essential gatherings
- avoiding common greetings, such as handshakes
- limiting contact with people at higher risk (e.g. older adults and those in poor health)
- keeping a distance of at least 2 arms lengths (approximately 2 metres) from others, as much as possible

Here's how you can practice social distancing:
- greet with a wave instead of a handshake, a kiss or a hug
- stay at home as much as possible, including for meals and entertainment
- shop or take public transportation during off-peak hours
- conduct virtual meetings
- host virtual playdates for your kids
- use technology to keep in touch with friends and family

If possible,
- use food delivery services or online shopping
- exercise at home or outside
- work from home

.

.

.

I have been practising social distancing for almost a year. The world is still. It is moving at my speed and I feel at home in it. The pandemic has given me wind.

.

.

.

Prime Minister Justin Trudeau[50]: "Listening is your duty and staying home is your way to serve."

.

.

.

I am this country's most faithful patriot.

~ ~ ~

.

I am listening to a new recording of Antonin Dvořák's Requiem in B minor, Op. 89. My tea should be ready. I have visited the Dvořák statue in front of the Rudolfinum in Prague.

.

.

.

My tea is ready.

.

.

.

"Mors stupebit, et natura,
Cum resurget creatura,
Judicanti responsura."[51]

Death and nature will marvel,
When the creature arises,
To respond to the Judge.

.

.

.

I have finished my tea.

~ ~ ~

"How to protect your mental health amid the outbreak"[52]

"While social distancing during this pandemic is hard on everyone, the stress and uncertainty can be particularly difficult for people with mental health disorders."

.

.

.

The world is still. It is moving at my speed and I feel at home in it.

.

.

.

"If you're gonna live, then live,
Don't talk about it."[53]

~ ~ ~

Suffering is present. Death is present. It is thrilling and I am neither suffering nor dead.

.

.

.

I haven't felt so good in months. In more than a year, really. I don't want it to end.

.

.

.

The pandemic has given me wind.

.

.

.

I don't owe you an explanation.

~ ~ ~

I'm no fool. I realize this is

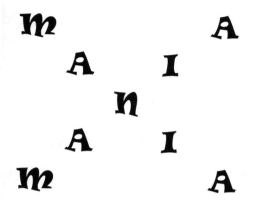

~ ~ ~

Or am I simply finding a way to be alone, separate?

~ ~ ~

"How To Protect Your Mental Health During The Coronavirus Pandemic, According To Psychologists"[54]

"If you've been feeling anxious, frustrated, angry or downright confused lately, know that you're not alone — we are all in this together."

.
.
.

I am calm, satisfied, pleased and downright clearheaded. And I know I am alone. I am in this all alone.

.
.
.

From one of the psychologists interviewed for the article: "If a person has pre-existing mental illness or history with anxiety and depression, it can often worsen and intensify during times such as these."

.
.
.

"...anxiety and depression..."

"...and..."

And?

Psychologists know nothing. Absolutely nothing. Nothing at all.

.

.

.

Foucault? Foucault knows.

"There is a very good reason why psychology can never master madness; it is because psychology became possible in our world only when madness had already been mastered and excluded from the drama. And when, in lightning flashes and cries, it reappears, as in Nerval or Artaud, Nietzsche or Roussel, it is psychology that remains silent, *speechless*, before this language that borrows a meaning from its own from that tragic split, from that freedom that, for contemporary man, only the existence of 'psychologists' allows him to forget."[55]

Mic drop.

.

.

.

"...excluded from the drama."

.

.

.

I couldn't care less about the "anxious, frustrated, angry and downright confused", about their "history". Not a jot. And they couldn't care less about me. I'd expect nothing less. I wouldn't want them to.

We're enemies, they and I. We despise each other. We loathe the weakness in each other and rarely talk about it. I wouldn't have it any other way, and neither would they. We are enemies.

When we pass on the street we don't look up or over to meet the other's eye. We keep on walking as if we were healthy and they were sick. We cannot look them in the eye and we wouldn't bother to do so if we could. They are a waste of our time, harmful even, and nothing, absolutely nothing in them is reflected in us, or vice versa. We are both of us excluded from the drama and there is no togetherness in exclusion.

So we keep on walking.

~ ~ ~

Pope Francis has requested that the faithful unite at noon CET tomorrow, March 25, the Feast of the Annunciation, to pray the "Our Father".

"Let us pray together for the sick, for the people who are suffering. We seek refuge under your protection, O Holy Mother of God. Do not despise our pleas — we who are put to the test — and deliver us from every danger. O glorious and blessed Virgin. I thank all Christians, all the men and women of goodwill who will pray at this moment, in unison, whichever religious tradition they belong to." #PrayForTheWorld[56]

.
.
.

"...O Holy Mother of God."

.
.
.

As he speaks this line in the video posted to Twitter, Francis is pictured praying in front of the *Salus Populi Romani* in the Borghese Chapel of the Basilica di Santa Maria Maggiore. I have a print of *Salus Populi Romani* and a rosary from the Basilica. The day after I was there, Pope Francis passed directly in front of me in St. Peter's Square.

.
.
.

Tomorrow I will do as he says.

.
.
.

"...we who are put to the test..."

~ ~ ~

Martha Higareda, the Mexican actor, posted a portion of Chapter 47 of the *Tao Te Ching*[57] to her Instagram account.

I like the first line: "No need to leave your door to know the whole world."

.

.

.

What will happen to me when all this is over?

.

.

.

"...when all this is over."

.

.

.

I don't have to tell you anything. We are not on the same side.

~ ~ ~

"They may have forbidden me to travel through a city, one place, but they left me the entire universe: infinity and eternity are at my command."[58]

~ ~ ~

The days are going by too quickly. I thought it was supposed to be the opposite during a pandemic. At least, that's what people tell me.

.

.

.

I'm concerned that things are backwards. What will happen to me when all this is over?

.

.

.

I felt very tired today.

.

.

.

"Run from me, darlin',
Run, my good wife.
Run from me, darlin',
You better run for your life."

~ ~ ~

I like these lines from a column today in *The Guardian*[59]: "The present is where we are and it's unsafe. Knowing this is one thing, feeling it another. The poet and novelist Rainer Maria Rilke knew about uncertainty. He told us to stop looking for answers and to learn to love the questions, 'like locked rooms and like books written in a foreign language.' We don't know what is going to happen."

.

.

.

"The present is where we are and it's unsafe."

.

.

.

What is going on here?

~ ~ ~

If you type "We Take" into Google, your browser will autofill "the Dead From Morning Till Night." The link is to a March 27, 2020 article in *The New York Times*, perhaps the most-read piece on the coronavirus to date.[60] Near the top of the page is a photograph taken by Fabio Bucciarelli. It shows a man—Claudio Travelli—lying in bed, wrapped in blankets with a cloth on his head. A Bergamo truck driver who contracted COVID-19 in early March, Sig. Travelli is being attended by two Red Cross workers who will shortly put him in an ambulance. The face of the first Red Cross volunteer is obscured, but the embroidered patch on his jacket stands out on the left of the picture. The second, holding a clipboard, is looking down at Sig. Travelli, who, himself, is looking to his left, at one of his daughters, who is looking back at him. A second daughter, at the right of the image, is looking across the scene to the first volunteer. She is looking at him, who is presumably looking at the second Red Cross worker, who is looking at Sig. Travelli, who is looking at his first daughter. And above his head, looking down on him, is an image of the Virgin Mary.

It's already a famous photograph. It's an almost perfect photograph. But I don't see suffering in it—or bravery or worry. I see an almost perfect photograph. I've already looked at it for quite a while. There's a harmony in the photograph that completely overwhelms whatever tragedy, whatever chaos or disharmony, there is in the situation it depicts. And I keep looking at the pulse oximeter on Sig. Travelli's right index finger. I wonder if it would have been what Barthes might have obsessed over as well.

Punctum.

.

.

.

"Do I contradict myself? Very well then, I contradict myself,
I am large — I contain multitudes."

.

.

.

"Help me make it through the night,
I don't care who's right or wrong.
I don't try to understand,
Let the devil take tomorrow,
Lord tonight I need a friend."

.

.

.

Early this evening, for a very brief time, I was very sad.

~ ~ ~

From today's *Winnipeg Free Press*, my local paper: "It's unexpectedly liberating. I feel like a brain in a jar. I feel unencumbered. I feel free."[61]

~ ~ ~

A headline from the April 3, 2020 edition of *The New York Times*: "Half the World Is Under Stay-Home Order; White House Debates Face Masks."[62] Is it that I find it comforting, the knowledge that "half the world" is now, and quite suddenly, at my level? I have experience here, in the mud. I am ahead of them, and they have complained more often and more loudly in the last few weeks than I have in the last 11 months, and the 13 years before that, and the bad time before that. Is it that I feel I'm better than them?

.

.

.

Even outdoors, in the rare outdoors, there are face masks, more and more of them each day. They are uniforms, badges, marks of the mud, emblems of the gross, the disgusting, of the disgusting creatures who wear them and who are tired of cooking, tired of using the toilet, tired of thinking. You can't see them. They are creatures of the mud, and mud is their home.

~ ~ ~

Is it that I find it comforting, the daily, sometimes hourly messages from the Prime Minister, the health officials, the broadcasters? "We will all get through this together." Is it comforting, the unexpected company and the sudden population of the mud, the reassurances that there are many of us here and that "we will all get through this" and that it will all come to an end? Will it come to an end for me as well? What will happen to me? What will become of me?

.

.

.

"What will become of me?"

.

.

.

Are you paying attention?

.

.

.

Do you understand?

~ ~ ~

Is it satisfying to have, even for just a little while, some company in the mud? Is it pleasing to have such regular reminders of their boredom, their loneliness, their despair? Is it enjoyable to watch the world writhe and hear it groan, to see it struggle and listen to it complain?

Yes, I think it is.

.

.

.

When this is over, what will become of me?

.

.

.

"When this is over..."

.

.

.

There is no interaction that isn't ultimately a wound.

.

.

.

"Yesterday is dead and gone,
And tomorrow's out of sight,
And it's sad to be alone."[63]

~ ~ ~

How do I tell them how my body feels?

The relentless discomfort of bloating. The pain in my neck and upper back that is causing me to stoop. A headache that comes and goes. The nighttime fevers. The overwhelming, devastating fatigue. So much of this is physical.

Do I have to tell them?

.

.

.

I am disgusting, a disgusting creature, mud is my home. You can't see me. I'm lying in mud and mud is my home.

~ ~ ~

It's already Wednesday in Wuhan, where the pandemic began[64], and the city has returned to work. "Returned to work" — that's the line we use. My city has been under a state of emergency for nearly three weeks. "Under" a state of emergency. I like that. It really does seem as though there is a weight from above bearing down and keeping everything "under" it in a state of pause, not so much frozen in time as in limbo, in motionless uncertainty. But when it's all over (...when it's all over...) the city will return to work. It will emerge, move, from "under" as there will be no overtop. It will "return to work". This city, this province, this country, "the west" (oh how I hate that term), the world will "return to work". That's what we've done with our time on this earth. When we halt, however briefly, the everything in the history of everything that has brought us to this moment, the most we can anticipate — indeed, the desire of the ages — is "Return-To-Work".

.

.

.

We are disgusting, disgusting creatures, mud is our home. You can't see us. We're lying in mud and mud is our home.

~ ~ ~

Is it because, while the world is doing next to nothing, I'm suddenly an achiever? There they are, cooped up and filthy, cutting their own hair; the lucky few who will never Return-To-Work because they never stopped are trudging in long, pathetic lines, single file, to the bus stop and a bus that smells of bleach, onward to industry, making and distributing the few things the wretched majority will need in their squalor; and I, achieving, look down on them, on those who are only now learning to wipe their asses with napkins and notebook paper, I am ahead of them, vibrant, smug, doing all sorts of productive things and cupping an ear for any sound of despair that will raise me up even higher above the newly despicable, their groans the fuel in my engine of industry.

.

.

.

"Return-To-Work..."

.

.

.

"Achieving..."

.

.

.

What will become of me when all this is over?

.

.

.

"...when all this is over..."

.
.
.

I don't owe you an explanation and I won't bear the balance of guilt.

~ ~ ~

"They may have forbidden me to travel through a city, one place, but they left me the entire universe: infinity and eternity are at my command."

~ ~ ~

A headline from the April 3, 2020 edition of *The Globe and Mail*: "Recessions might actually be good for your health."[65]

A few lines from the article: "Suicides do go up in recessions. However, in every other respect, the evidence indicates that recessions are actually good for your health. On average, during a downturn people eat better, drink less and exercise more (maybe they're keeping themselves ready for their next job interview?). There are fewer accidents on the job, fewer deaths on the road and, as just about everybody who lives in a city has noticed these past few weeks, we breathe cleaner air since emissions drop."

None of this is news to me, although I'm curious about the author's almost thrown-away line, bracketed as if it was meant to be some sort of upbeat aside. Are we using this period of quiet and enforced inactivity to merely wait to "return to normal", to Return-To-Work? If so, what a waste! And it's especially a waste given that this respite, this jubilee, is being borne by the backs of workers whose toil continues even now. What better time—perhaps the only time in our lives—to have a good, hard think about them and about ourselves and about everyone and then, "when this is all over", to have done something about it.

Of course, there are parents going crazy with children at home instead of school, others for whom home was never a safe place and is even more dangerous now, the families whose lives have been ruined by this pandemic. They have so little energy to do something about anything, to even think. I almost pity them. But I don't. If I said I did I'd be lying. They never cared about me, noticed me. They never looked me in the eye and I was a ghost among them. No longer. Now they are ghosts, and we are even.

.

.

.

What is going on here?

~ ~ ~

I interviewed for a job yesterday. On Zoom.[66] Most people would say it's a good job. I "did well", they told me. I suppose I smiled at the right times and leaned back in my chair with the right amount of confidence. I have learned to act and have many years of acting experience. Today the recruiter sent me an email suggesting that I write the employer a "thank-you note". To thank them for what, exactly? For speaking with me? For needing me to do something for them? For giving me "this exciting opportunity and thank-you very much for your time, sir, I just want to get my foot in the door, sir, I'm going to get it in some door and I'm selective about doors but I have a good feeling about this door, sir"?

.

.

.

"All I want to do is walk straight out the door. Mid-sentence. Just get up, boy. Stop talking and stop shooting this junk out of your mouth and head out the door mid-sentence. Give them the last thing they'd ever expect. Just when they're getting a feel for me and really getting into it and leaning back and really getting the feel on and giving me their daughter's phone number. Just when they're imagining the day they hand me the keys. Right when they're thinking that this young man is just like me 30 years ago and taking a shot for a foot in the door. Right then, boy. Get up and give them what they'd least expect and walk out the door. Right when they think they know you and what you really want and how sincere it all sounds from your junk-shooting mouth. Get up, boy. When you go home tonight and take stock of the things you have, know that this is not how you want to have those things. This is not how you want to make a life for yourself. So get up, boy, and walk out that door. Let them stop leaning and be all flustered that the young man could walk out mid-sentence. Even if they're the only ones who ever know that it's not good enough for you to sit there and blow junk out of your mouth and come back every day for the rest of your life to blow more junk. Let them know it. Just when they think they have you. Blow them away and let them know that what they have is not good enough for you."

.

.

.

I wrote those last lines almost exactly 14 years ago. I'm not so young anymore. And I ended up blowing junk out of my mouth for 13 years. Then, like Nietzsche's clock, it all fell apart.

.

.

.

But it's never too late to get the hell out of there, to walk out mid-sentence and give them what they'd least expect. To tell them and yourself that you're done. Finished. Especially when a global pandemic has done you the biggest favour of the last 14 years.

.

.

.

I replied to the recruiter to let him know I would not be accepting the job. After all, I did not receive a thank-you note from the employer.

.

.

.

I'm done. Finished. I want out and I am out. Done.

~ ~ ~

"Do I contradict myself? Very well then, I contradict myself, I am large — I contain multitudes."

~ ~ ~

Because of the closures[67], there is nowhere within walking distance that I can get a cappuccino. That's my biggest worry today.

.
.
.

"Run from me, darlin',
Run, my good wife.
Run from me, darlin',
You better run for your life."

.
.
.

What is going on here?

.
.
.

I don't have to tell you anything.

.
.
.

We are not on the same side.

~ ~ ~

From the April 10, 2020 edition of *The New York Times*[68]: "I know I am not the only one thinking these thoughts. Perhaps this isolation will finally give people the chance to do what writers do: imagine, empathize, dream. To have the time and luxury to do these things is already to live on the edge of utopia, even if what writers often do from there is to imagine the dystopic. I write not only because it brings me pleasure, but also out of fear — fear that if I do not tell a new story, I cannot truly live."

.

.

.

"...imagine, empathize, dream."

I'm well-versed in all three. And yes, even empathy. Though not at the moment. My empathy is worn down, like the lead in a pencil it no longer makes sense to sharpen, like the soles of shoes that have done too much walking.

Besides, they tell me I'm "not feeling right" about the pandemic, about the shuttering of the economy and the social isolation. I am a "sociopath" because I'm getting things done and making the most of my time, of this precious time, of this invaluable time when I'm achieving and they're not, when I'm making sense of the world and they're at a loss, when my thoughts are sharp and theirs have dulled.

They also told me I wasn't "feeling right" when everything was "normal", so I'm quite finished with their analyses. And yes, my empathy is worn down.

It'll be back, don't worry. But only when they've earned it. I understand that such a statement goes against the spirit of empathy, but that's just how it's going to be for a bit. And they'll earn it, don't worry. Just not yet. They have more to repay to me first.

.

.

.

"I know I am not the only one thinking these thoughts."

~ ~ ~

There is still so much I'm not telling you.

~ ~ ~

From an Al Jazeera article entitled "Will coronavirus signal the end of capitalism?"[69] by Paul Mason: "Left-wing economists, myself included, have been warning that, in the long term, stagnant growth and high debt were likely to lead to these three policies: States paying citizens a universal income as automation makes well-paid work precarious and scarce; central banks lending directly to the state to keep it afloat; and large-scale public ownership of major corporations maintaining vital services that cannot be run at a profit."

And, a bit further down: "But now, the unthinkable is here — all of it: Universal payments, state bailouts and the funding of state debts by central banks have all been adopted at a speed that has shocked even the usual advocates of these measures."

.

.

.

I've wanted to unpack this for a few days, but I needed a better brand of tea first. Now I have it.

By Appointment to
HRH The Prince of Wales
Suppliers of Beverages, Taylors of Harrogate
North Yorkshire

The inside of the box is a lovely white and blue wallpaper-style pattern. Also, we've known that automation required accompanying universal income for more than 170 years. The failure to accelerate technology and socialism in tandem was one of the great failures of the 20th century. And even if the "three policies" are temporary, I find their presence rather funny. Universal income: a hearty chuckle. Central banks lending to the state: a fit of laughter. Large-scale public ownership of major corporations: ROTFL.[70]

.

.

.

I'm enjoying this tea.

~ ~ ~

Please don't judge me too harshly. I've been inside for almost a year. I don't know what's going to happen.

.
.
.

"Solitude gives birth to the original in us, to beauty unfamiliar and perilous — to poetry. But also, it gives birth to the opposite: to the perverse, the illicit, the absurd."[71]

.
.
.

"I don't know what's going to happen."

.
.
.

I went for a walk this afternoon. I passed a school sign that read "Learning Suspended Indefinitely" as well as three horcruxes.

.
.
.

This is not a novel.

~ ~ ~

I read a newspaper column this morning, but I don't want to reference it in the usual way. I'm going to quote one or two lines of it, though. It's really bad. Two lines—I just decided to include the second one. I don't want to give the author any additional attention, but I guess I have to include a proper reference in the endnotes. You can look there if you must. Generally, I hope you're looking up the endnotes. I know it's a pain in the ass, but I think some of the references in these pages are really neat, and I wonder if you might think the same. Anyway, enough delaying.

"Yet, as always, at the bottom of depression's box there is hope."[72]

What the actual what?

There are four problems with that sentence, and that doesn't include the "Yet", which, if you read the previous paragraph (don't) makes absolutely no sense whatsoever. Number one: "...as always..." As what "always"? As the "classic case"? As the outlined, defined, common-knowledge "pathology"? As the "of course I recognise this, I've seen it a million times" "always"? Spare me. Number two: "...at the bottom..." Serenity now. The assumption of "bottom" as an identifiable surface, as anything but hindsight, is preposterous. Moving on. Number three: "...of depression's box..." The author has given himself away there. What, pray tell, is he putting in the box? The "classic cases"? There's also the assumption, if you read the entire column (don't), that the author and other fortunates have climbed out of the box and can thus peer down on the lessers within, "at the bottom". More often than not, boxes are a metaphorical no-no. But, and this is the part where you throw up in your mouth, this box does, indeed, contain something. And what does it contain? Why, "hope", of course! Number four: "...there is hope". Hope in a box. And not just any box. "Depression's box." A box with a "bottom". "As always."

The second line: "I feel singularly well-placed to comfort those who are taking their first deep plunge into depression."

Look, maybe I just don't get the style—the writing style, the medical style. Fair enough. That's my deal. And I do like the use of "comfort" in this sentence. But the arrogance, the positioning of expertise is something from which I immediately, almost instinctively, recoil. Again, my deal. I'm just not one for pop psychology. It may very well emanate from a sincere experience or place, but when it morphs into "singularly well-placed" self-help tips masquerading as expertise, I'm just not interested. Look, even Peter Youngren saves souls. I'd just rather be somewhere else while he's doing it.

.
.
.

Congrats on the house upstate, by the way. Thumbs up.

.
.
.

Foucault, once again, can take it from here.

"There is a very good reason why psychology can never master madness; it is because psychology became possible in our world only when madness had already been mastered and excluded from the drama. And when, in lightning flashes and cries, it reappears, as in Nerval or Artaud, Nietzsche or Roussel, it is psychology that remains silent, *speechless* before this language that borrows a meaning from its own from that tragic split, from that freedom that, for contemporary man, only the existence of 'psychologists' allows him to forget."[73]

.

.

.

Foucault in the face.

.

.

.

I don't owe you an explanation and I won't bear the balance
of guilt.

~ ~ ~

Today my body quit at 6:00 p.m. Just quit. Stopped. It's not unusual, although it hasn't happened in a while. My teeth have been aching as well. I've been grinding my teeth at night. And my temples ache. Likely because of my teeth. My eyes hurt. So much of this is physical.

.

.

.

I know that this will one day kill me.

~ ~ ~

Underlying my reaction, I think, is the knowledge that it's not COVID-19 that made me sick. It's not COVID-19 that will kill me.

.

.

.

"…the world had become 'silent, icy, dead'…"

~ ~ ~

Yesterday my car wouldn't start. It's only now that I can write about it. Everything was thrown off because it wouldn't start. Such seems to be the tenuousness of my state that a single unexpected or inconvenient event can throw everything off and ruin a day. Now, I'll admit that even being "thrown off" or "having a day ruined" is a luxury and not something I would have experienced even a few weeks ago. That's progress. But it also reveals the delicacy of my state, and I didn't realise how delicate it was. I've been following a very strict schedule, and for many weeks that schedule has been undisturbed. Until yesterday. I felt dizzy. My appetite vacillated and my stomach was unsettled. I was useless. There was no helping it. I can't function with an upset stomach. Nietzsche was right about the stomach.

.

.

.

Are you paying attention?

.

.

.

Are you hopscotching?

.

.

.

Do you understand?

~ ~ ~

"Get lost, madame, get up off my knee
Keep your mouth away from me
I'll keep the path open, the path in my mind
I'll see to it that there's no love left behind
I'll play Beethoven's sonatas, and Chopin's preludes
I contain multitudes."[74]

.

.

.

I much prefer Chopin's nocturnes. Who doesn't?

.

.

.

How do you know I'm not writing another book at the same time I'm writing this one? Like, a parallel manuscript. You don't. You don't know anything. You only know what I want you to know. I am the Minister of Information. I am large — I contain multitudes.

.

.

.

This is a novel and the other book is the real book.

.

.

.

My stomach is unsettled.

~ ~ ~

"The Serpent that announces, 'The World is a closed thing, cyclical, resonant, eternally-returning,' is to be delivered into a system whose only aim is to violate the Cycle."[75]

.
.
.

"...a trauma, a trauma..."

~ ~ ~

For years, for more than a decade, I have ignored them. The Blue Journals. Four of them, stacked neatly one on top of the other, at the bottom of a bookshelf, other things resting on them, stacking up, dusty, unread. Today I picked them up, wiped off the dust, and read all four. Read them for the first time. They are from the erased part, the missing part, the penmanship is exceptional. I read them to find out if I remembered anything. I didn't. The erasing was thorough.

.

.

.

The Blue Journals oscillate from bitterness to desperation. They are beautiful, although of course I'd say that. I wrote them. Supposedly. I have them and I've had them since they were written, so I might as well have written them. The penmanship is exceptional, the account of desolation a scratch, a wound. I have the scars, so I must have written them.

.

.

.

An entry from the Blue Journals:

"I can't sleep at night. There is a floor-to-ceiling window near my bed and I am terrified of it when I lie awake in bed. I roll away from it and turn my back to it but I know it is there and it terrifies me and I can't sleep for anything. Sometimes I forget the window and almost fall asleep. But something nudges me awake and reminds me of the window and I lie in bed and cannot fall asleep. I think it is God nudging me. It is not enough that he trips up my every step and makes a shambles out of my life during the day. It is not enough for him unless he can also disturb my sleep and keep my body from resting."

And on the next page:

"I've been writing about myself and about my thoughts as if I'll be leaving them to someone as an explanation. So things make sense to them and my behaviour makes sense and what they might think is bad luck makes sense to them."

Then, about suicide:

"When I think about it now, it is calmer and more peaceful and more rational in my head. It is an option."

.

.

.

There is mystery in the Blue Journals, a reference to something of which I have no memory, not that I remember anything about the time of the Blue Journals, but it's a reference to something I should have, an item in my possession. I do not have it. I have been looking for it but I cannot find it.

The reference: "He might read the letter that he saved."

What letter? Exactly what letter am I talking about? Supposing that it was I who wrote that line, which letter might I have read? And what did it say? If I saved it, assuming it was for me and addressed to me, had I already read it at least once? Or had I saved it to read later? And what might "later" have meant? What might I have been thinking about when I thought of "later", the time when I "might read the letter"?

I think I know who wrote the letter, assuming it was a letter addressed to me and that I knew at the time who had written it and it was, indeed, I who referenced it in the notebook I allegedly filled with writing, part of a series of notebooks I keep on a shelf, propping up other items, a series I purportedly wrote during a period of which I have no recollection. I am like Yambo at the house in Solara,[76] searching for things that might tell me who I was, might explain who I became, going through odds and ends and music and books to piece myself together, looking in vain for a letter I once had but have no longer.

Did I throw it away? Did I hide it somewhere? Is it lingering, flattened by years and the weight of other things, at the bottom of a drawer or in a box in the closet? Was it lost? Perhaps in a moving van or in the process of moving from one place to another? I rather doubt it. If it was important enough to be referenced as "saved", "the letter that he saved", then surely it would have been kept well and protected, at least while he had it, which he no longer does. At least he can't find it. If he threw it away, burned it or shredded it or sent it down the chute with the garbage, what would have caused him to do so? What would he have been feeling when he parted with it, with this "saved" thing? Was he sad, upset? Maybe crying or hurt or even devastated? Might he have laughed, or smiled to himself? Would he have felt nothing at all?

What answers might the letter have contained? Or questions. Phrases. Voice. Emotion. Nostalgia. Was it so important, so secretive that I referred to it as a "saved" thing?

Could it have been the most important thing in my life?

.

.

.

"I have been looking for it but I cannot find it."

~ ~ ~

"Recounting an event distorts it, recounting facts distorts and twists and almost negates them, everything that one recounts, however true, becomes unreal and approximate, the truth doesn't depend on things actually existing or happening, but on their remaining hidden or untold."[77]

.

.

.

"...on their remaining hidden or untold."

~ ~ ~

"We were dancin' all night
Then they took you away — stole you out of my life
You just need to remember"[78]

~ ~ ~

"Which of us, walking through the twilight or retracing some day in our past, has never felt that we have lost some infinite thing?"[79]

.
.
.

Are you paying attention?

.
.
.

Do you understand?

~ ~ ~

I have started reading a novel. I haven't read a novel in more than three months, maybe longer. It was a Patrick Modiano novel, and I read it in a couple days. But today I sat outside and began *My Brilliant Friend* by Elena Ferrante. I bought it yesterday, over the phone, and then picked it up outside the bookstore. We can't go into bookstores, but the booksellers can leave our purchases on the sidewalk or on a wooden ledge, which is where I got mine. I read it outside for a while and enjoyed it, but then I wanted to go inside. Thinking about going inside made me feel glad. It gave me the feeling that there were friends inside, waiting for me, even though I knew there was no one inside. It was books that I was thinking about, the books that stand in piles on either side of my computer, books to be touched and to be asked what they're thinking about. "Hello Roland, what's on your mind?" "Umberto, what's going on in that head of yours?" "Jorge, you tell one helluva story. Can you tell me another?" "Javier, what were you telling me the other day about memory?" "Just cut to the chase, Marcel."

Three months or more is a long time to go without reading a novel. I must have been busy with something. I can't remember what. That, or I just felt like sitting in the quiet. Yes, I must have just felt like sitting in the quiet.

.
.
.

I don't remember.

.
.
.

I don't owe an explanation.

.
.
.

What is going on here?

~ ~ ~

A tweet from the city police department: "Officers are currently in the area searching for an escaped prisoner. Many police units are on scene and we ask people to remain indoors while we search for the individual."

I want to go to my balcony and cheer! Let's all go outside at 7:00 p.m. and cheer for the prisoner![80] Cheer him on and into freedom! For this is a Time of Jubilee!

.

.

.

From Leviticus 25:8: "It shall be a jubilee for you; each one of you is to return to his family property and each to his own clan."

Sound the trumpet!

.

.

.

Leviticus 28: 13: "In this Year of Jubilee everyone is to return to his own property."

Sound the trumpet!

.

.

.

Leviticus 28:35: "If one of your countrymen becomes poor and is unable to support himself among you, help him as you would an alien or a temporary resident, so he can to continue to live among you."

Sound the trumpet!

"Jubilee," says the *Oxford Dictionary*, derives from the Late Latin *jubilaeus*, which itself derives from the Hebrew *yōḇēl* — a trumpet made of a ram's horn. The horn, or shofar, would be blown to announce the jubilee.

Sound the shofar!

Break chains! Forgive! Absolve! Annul! Live well and tread lightly! Love! Befriend! Enjoy! Feast together! Aid! Relieve! Affirm! Live generously! Release! Deliver! Emancipate! Declare goodness and sing of it! Dance!

"…Opens prison doors, sets the captives free…"[81]

From *The New York Times*' live website updates on April 26: "Prisons have become powerful breeding grounds for the coronavirus, prompting governments to release hundreds of thousands of inmates in a scramble to curb the spread of the contagion behind bars."

.

.

.

From Human Rights Watch's COVID-19 checklist on April 14, 2020: "Is your government releasing people who should not be in custody, including most pretrial detainees, people held for minor offenses, detainees who have not been charged, and non-violent juvenile offenders?...Are authorities considering for release prisoners at greater risk of serious illness from the virus, including older people, people with underlying health conditions, people with disabilities, and pregnant people?...Has your government released political prisoners and others wrongfully or arbitrarily imprisoned, including human rights defenders, journalists and political activists?...Has your government told its police forces to stop arrests of sex workers, non-violent drug offenders, people arrested for 'moral crimes,' and others who should not face criminal punishment, to avoid adding to crowded jails?"

.

.

.

There is so much I want to leave behind, to leave in the old world, in the before time, pre-pandemic. I want to forgive and be forgiven, absolve and be absolved, befriend and be a friend, declare goodness and sing of it, dancing. The old world isn't coming back, and I want to go out to my balcony and cheer. I want to applaud its exit and my freedom, to watch what I've left with it pass away with the old world, to die.

Sound the shofar!

.

.

.

A tweet from the city police department: "Update: The escaped prisoner has been taken into custody. We thank the public for their assistance."

.

.

.

When this is over, what will become of me?

.

.

.

"When this is over…"

~ ~ ~

From the April 26 edition of *The New York Times*[82]: "In the coming months, all of us are going to have to figure out how to gird ourselves psychologically for whatever the new normal might be. 'Optimism tempered by realism,' tends to be the favored formulation, and sure, that's fine; it may even be politically and economically sound."

The writer of the article is, of course, referencing the lockdowns resulting from the COVID-19 pandemic.

She continues: "But I'd also like to make a positive case for pessimism. Defensive pessimism, specifically. Because if things start going downhill, defensive pessimists will be the ones with their feet already on the brakes."

So far, so good. I'd agree with that, I'd even identify with it, as would a lot of other people. There's nothing particularly special, even rare, about defensive pessimism, which basically involves less a vigilance for worst-case scenarios than a bracing for them, a defence, all the while asserting control over what is controllable, such as mundane tasks or chores and near-term events. It's a mindset I'd think is quite common among Millennials, such as myself and, presumably, the writer of the article. In fact, the self-care industry depends on it.

Why am I going through this article? Because of where the writer takes it, and the casual, albeit oblivious, damage she inflicts on readers like me.

Her definition of defensive pessimists: "They are people who lean way back into their anxiety, rather than repress it or narcotize it or allow it to petrify them into stone."

Now, I'm all for leaning way back into anxiety, into exploring what's happening in such moments, but there is no such thing as "repressing" it. She's trying to praise herself here, as one of the brave, martyred, unmedicated sufferers of anxiety, and of pessimism, although the two aren't even close to the same thing, even if they often happen to go hand in hand. But it's the phrase "or narcotize it" that really makes this column irredeemable.

The *Merriam-Webster Dictionary* points out that "to narcotize" is "to treat with or subject to a narcotic" or "to put into narcosis." And "narcosis" is "a state of stupor, unconsciousness, or arrested activity produced by the influence of narcotics or other chemical or physical agents." Narcotics — and I like *Merriam-Webster's* second definition: "something that soothes, relieves or lulls" — are serious business, serious treatments for serious ailments. Neither they nor their consumers should be trivialised (such trivialisation is a direct cause of harm), and then there is the matter of the writer's link of pessimism to narcotics as a relief of that pessimism. What absolute nonsense! Suggesting narcotics as a treatment for pessimism — which isn't a condition — is right up there with prescribing the injection of disinfectants to cure coronavirus.[83]

I've had this article tab open on my web browser for three days and it still makes me angry. Because then she goes and says the "D" word. Of course she says the "D" word...

"In general, it is probably worth noting that depressives tend to be the true realists, not happy people."

I sincerely hope the writer isn't identifying as a "depressive," and no doubt one who eschews treatment and "represses" the symptoms of what is a serious illness, but I get the impression she is, as she goes on to describe "depressives" as "true realists, not happy people" — a similarly sloppy brushstroke to the one she applies over "anxiety", "pessimism" and treatment by narcotics. The thing is, her article would function perfectly well without linking "anxiety" and "depressives" to repression and rejection of treatment. Pessimism can certainly be a beneficial disposition during unsettling times,

times when it seems the world is actually falling apart. It can be beneficial, generally. But the careless references to and tie-ins with anxiety, depression and medication come across as self-serving, as if the writer is saying, as so many others do, "I've been there, I've got it too, I have 'the mental illnesses' and look how funny I am in spite of 'the mental illnesses', how clever I am, the loveable martyr." What's worse, readers at vulnerable periods of their actual illnesses will read this (well, hopefully not) and other items like it and recoil, sometimes dangerously, at the haphazard, belittling use of language and terminology. Writing such as this, either on its own or aggregated with similar content, can cause sickness to worsen, can even cause death.

Midway through the article, the writer talks about an online quiz she took that "qualified" her "as a defensive pessimist". I've just taken the quiz as well. My score is "72", whatever that means. Apparently I qualify as a defensive pessimist as well. Great? Really, though, who cares. So what. If I took the quiz a week from now my results might be totally different. Who cares. None of this is useful, and all of it causes more harm than good.

Take your meds, kids.

.

.

.

I can't wait to close this tab.

.

.

.

I've closed it.

We're enemies, they and I. We despise each other. We loathe the weakness in each other and rarely talk about it. I wouldn't have it any other way, and neither would they. We are enemies. Nothing in them is reflected in us, or vice versa. We are both of us excluded from the drama and there is no togetherness in exclusion.

.

.

.

We keep on walking.

.

.

.

Are you paying attention?

~ ~ ~

They are talking about reopening. Today my province will unveil its plan to "reopen the economy",[84] as popular parlance puts it. They'll provide the plan to Return-To-Work.

.

.

.

I'm not ready.

.

.

.

"...what will become of me?"

~ ~ ~

They are going to start reopening the economies in France, Italy, and Spain. Many Canadian provinces have already announced similar plans. This distresses me. I am not ready. The world has slowed to my speed and all the effort, all the energy, all the strength I exert to keep myself safe in the world has been legislated by the world and I'm not ready for that legislation to be lifted. The world finally works for me, makes sense for me. My days are full and the days are too short. I've started a Communication Science course through the University of Amsterdam. I read and walk and go to my Italian grocer and grind good coffee, I eat well and read some more and write and work and sit on my balcony, I watch the empty streets and listen to the birds and watch the daily mass on television, I have not missed the mass in more than a month. I have confessed my sins and done my time and now it is time for the world to repay me, to repay what it owes. There has not yet been enough suffering, not enough death. I have done my time and now the world is doing its time. And time isn't up. Not just yet. I'm not ready.

.

.

.

The world is a contagion, and I am my own parasite. I am disgusting, a disgusting creature, mud is my home.

.

.

.

When this is over, what will become of me?

.

.

.

"When this is over…"

~ ~ ~

I was quite tired today, and even now, as I write these words, I pause often and drop my forehead into the palms of my hands. I am very tired. It is a total fatigue, body and mind, and my body hurts and my head is heavy and exhausted. My back aches, so does my chest, I feel bloated, constipated. I should take a shower. I rarely bathe or shower, it's too much effort, removing clothes and getting into the shower and standing there, tired, and then moving my arms to wash my body and my hair, eyes heavy, rinsing, getting out of the shower and using my arms to dry my body and my hair with a towel, putting on clothes, deciding what to do next, collapsing into a chair.

.

.

.

How do I tell them how my body feels?

.

.

.

So much of this is physical.

.

.

.

"To each his own rhythm of suffering."[85]

~ ~ ~

I am so very tired. I sleep straight through the night without waking up and fall asleep quickly, but then in the morning I get out of bed and am tired, so very tired, as if the night was exhausting and the daytime the time to sleep, but then I would be always asleep, although I go through the day almost sleeping, short of temper, irritated by a fatigue that weighs on my body and presses against my brain, I can't concentrate and I fall asleep, but this time a terrifying sleep, tortured by hot white, yellow and red blazes of unrelenting light, asleep but not sleeping, dreaming but not dreaming, and then I wake up and am tired, so very tired, I am short of temper and irritated by everyone and everything, a voice, the room temperature, distance between myself and what must have been my aspirations when I was awake, really awake, and my head drops to my chest in exhaustion, my neck unfairly burdened and my back aching, my legs aching, my arms aching, no appetite, no anything, not even nothing, nothing would be better, nothing at all and the rest, the rest, the rest of nothing.

.

.

.

What is happening?

~ ~ ~

There is a dream I remember from my childhood. I was very young, perhaps five or six, and I dreamt I was in a sort of shop. There was a shelf not far from the counter and I was examining the things on the shelf. I don't remember what sort of things, but they must have been attractive things, desirable things, and then I realised the only light in the shop was from a small candle. The shopkeeper, an old, stooped man with scraggly white hair and a hollow face, was holding the candle, and he approached me. He came right up to me and looked at me with his terrifying face, and then, teeth grinding as he sneered at me, he blew out the candle.

.

.

.

"...two rhythms are in some manner running at once..."[86]

.

.

.

Are you paying attention?

.

.

.

Do you understand?

~ ~ ~

There are times when I'm very aware that I am alone.

.

.

.

I look out my living room window, and there is no one. I look to the street, and there is no one. I am so very tired and I am the only one here. I am so very tired and I am the only one here and there is only guilt. Everything is guilt and fatigue. I am tired and because I am so very tired I am guilty, and I am guilty because I'm tired, so very tired.

.

.

.

"At bottom, and just in the deepest and most important things, we are unutterably alone..."[87]

.

.

.

There are times when I'm very aware that I am alone.

~ ~ ~

What am I?

Tired.

How tired am I?

So very tired.

.

.

.

Are you paying attention?

~ ~ ~

"Help me make it through the night
I don't care who's right or wrong
I don't try to understand
Let the devil take tomorrow
Lord tonight I need a friend
Yesterday is dead and gone
And tomorrow's out of sight
And it's sad to be alone."[88]

~ ~ ~

Soon it will be summer. The days are long and the evenings are bright and mild. I just came in from the balcony, where I was drinking my tea and reading a book. Did I do this last spring and summer, or even in the autumn, until it was too cold to sit outside? Did I read outside with a cup of tea in the bright, warm evening? I don't remember. The piles of books on my desk, unshelved and ascending like my own, personal Babel, suggest I did, but I don't remember.

Not for the first time, there will be a chunk of months, a year more or less, that simply won't have happened, that won't have lodged in my memory, memories that take up space. Others may tell me about that time, but likely not in the near term, they remember it well and it wasn't easy for them. For a while we'll all pretend it didn't happen, although for me it didn't, I have scars to show but I don't know where I got them, perhaps I'll invent a retason, a memory, a memory to take up space, a memory of a memory, recounting an event distorts it, Javier Marias wrote that "...the truth doesn't depend on things actually existing or happening, but on their remaining hidden or unknown or untold".[89] He also wrote that "We cannot know what time will do to us with its fine, indistinguishable layers upon layers, we cannot know what it might make of us."

.

.

.

I have layers missing. I can feel the gaps into which my memory bends.

.

.

.

I suppose I have these pages, although I'll never read them. I don't remember writing most of them. You'll have to remind me. If you paid attention. If you understood.

I can do that. But will it really help?

It must.

Why?

Because I can't think of anything else that will.

I guess it's worth a shot.

It has to be.

Can I ask you something?

Of course.

Why do you want to be reminded? Wouldn't it better to not remember, to just forget and move on?

It would be easier. Maybe even better. But it's not what I want.

Why?

Because I want to know who I am. I want to know about the things that have made me. I don't have to like them, I don't have to feel anything toward those things, but I want to know about them. Knowing what has made us is part of being human, and if I don't know, if I forget, the next time this happens I'll have trouble staying in a body that can't make sense of itself, that hurts.

Why do you say, "the next time"?

Because there will be a next time.

How do you know?

Because there have already been several times, and when it happens again I want to know about it, I don't want any surprises, I want a memory that takes up space.

Then I shall remind you. I will refresh your memory.

How?

By living and being gentle. Isn't that what you wanted?

I think so.

Did you forget?

I'm already fading.

.
.
.

"There's a gap in between
There's a gap where we meet
Where I end and you begin...
...I can watch but not take part"[90]

.
.
.

"Run from me darlin'"

~ ~ ~

"I note that Some — gone patient long —
At length, renew their smile —
An imitation of a Light
That has so little Oil"[91]

~ ~ ~

Good energy frightens me. At the very least I am wary of it, suspicious, distrustful of the vitality, the productivity, worried that it is yet another trick, a false dawn, a ruse that will convince me and satisfy others before abandoning me in an instant, or during the night's sleep, grinding its teeth and sneering before blowing out the candle. It is a dread that runs constantly in the background, like an application on a mobile phone, invisible, yet spending the battery's power and sapping energy. There is no purely good energy because of that application, one I didn't install, I wasn't consulted, and yet I can't close it, can't restart, the best I can do is not think about it, about the good energy, and prepare as best I can for the application to reveal itself as a virus, I am my own pet virus, to be glad for just a moment that the energy is good, and then to prepare for the virus, the pouring in and cold and sweating and spreading, the sickness, so old a pain.

There is the one glad moment and then I prepare. I sleep so as to charge the battery and prevent the application from gaining overwhelming power. I eat so as to diminish the energy and weigh me down, filling my body with heaviness that might weaken the energy and avert the trick, or at least forestall it. I calculate my presentations, appearing only in the glad moments and escaping when suspicion mounts. I am the Minister of Information. The rest of the time I keep to myself, wrapped in the comfort that I am also made of things that didn't happen. [92]

This is what I would consider a good day, a good bit of life, good energy as I understand it, even if I know there is more, so much more, I can see it around me and in others, but it's a good day for me, and as I peer into that pond, primordial, the embryonic sea, I witness, as though I were finally seeing the hidden thing, the flickering reflection of my desires.[93]

Oh, to bathe in it. Oh, to drink of it.

Not yet.

.
.
.

Are you paying attention?

.
.
.

Do you understand?

~ ~ ~

"A broken and contrite spirit
Thou wilt not despise."

Psalm 57:17

Suicide note of the writer Richard Barham Middleton.

~ ~ ~

Afterword

Jerrad got quite sick after finishing this manuscript. He had a lot of people worried, and I'll just add that it was touch and go for a bit there. He wanted me to pass that along, and of course I said that I would. He also insisted that I leave this afterword unsigned so as not to be "implicated". I told him his request made no sense and that I was happy to sign my name to it, but he was adamant. He was admittedly paranoid. Finally, he requested that I say that he's sorry. He wanted to write through the summer and fall, but the pandemic and series of lockdowns that so buoyed him in the spring finally ground him down. He says he doesn't remember anything of August, and I believe him. He doesn't exaggerate things like that.

In exchange for honouring his wishes I asked for a few lines of licence, which he readily granted.

These are some difficult pages to read, for me anyway. This isn't the Jerrad I'm familiar with, and I think that's exactly the point. He wants me, wants us, to see him as he sometimes is, not just as the friend I'm fortunate to know. He has occasionally told me that when he experiences an episode, particularly an extended one, he doesn't want anyone to look at him. I think what he's done here is asked us to look at him after the fact, when the intensity has subsided somewhat. "Are you paying attention?" For me it's a question of urgency. "Do you understand?" A plea. Like I said, he doesn't exaggerate these things.

The Jerrad I know is gentle and kind. I enjoy interacting with him. Sometimes I think he wrote this book for me, as if he's showing me the parts he hides so I see him as whole. It's an honest endeavour. To conclude, I'd like to share a short poem he texted me the other day, when we went back and forth over what my part in this would look like.

My heart breaks every day
Is it too much
What did Trent Reznor say
The only thing that's real
But I remember everything
Come here and let me touch
No way
Hurts too damn much

Endnotes

1   *Hopscotch*, by Julio Cortázar, is a novel that can be read in both linear and prescribed sequence.

2   Gandalf's words to Pippin ahead of the Battle of the Pelennor Fields, from *The Lord of the Rings: The Return of the King*, by J.R.R. Tolkien.

3   An entry from *Letters to a Young Poet*, by Rainer Maria Rilke.

4   Lyrics from "Milk It", by Kurt Cobain and Nirvana.

5   "I seal that which was not to be said in the tomb that I become" is a line from *The Name of the Rose*, by Umberto Eco.

6   A reference to *The Library of Babel*, by Jorge Luis Borges.

7   An entry from *Malone Dies*, by Samuel Beckett.

8   An entry from *My Brilliant Friend*, by Elena Ferrante.

9   Lyrics from "Milk It", by Kurt Cobain and Nirvana.

10   An entry from *The Notebooks of Malte Laurids Brigge*, by Rainer Maria Rilke.

11   A quote attributed to Thomas Jefferson.

12   An entry from *Mourning Diary*, by Roland Barthes.

13   An entry from *A Heart So White*, by Javier Marias.

14   An entry from *Gravity's Rainbow*, by Thomas Pynchon.

15   Paul Valery, from his essay, "Variations on Eclogues".

16   An entry from *The Pleasure of the Text*, by Roland Barthes.

17   *The Origin of the Work of Art*, by Martin Heidegger.

18   The painting "A Pair of Shoes", by Vincent van Gogh.

19   An entry from *Tonio Kroger*, by Thomas Mann.

20   Cited in *Madness and Civilization*, by Michel Foucault.

21   An entry from *Ecce Homo*, by Friedrich Nietzsche.

22   Lyrics from "Milk It", by Kurt Cobain and Nirvana.

23   Lyrics from "Happy", by Julia Michaels.

24   An entry from *Young Once*, by Patrick Modiano.

25   An entry from *The Trial*, by Franz Kafka.

26   An entry from *Mourning Diary*, by Roland Barthes.

27   Spanish-language television series that debuted on Telecinco and was later picked up by Netflix.

28   An entry from *Camera Lucida*, by Roland Barthes.

29   An entry from *Mourning Diary*, by Roland Barthes.

30   An entry from *Camera Lucida*, by Roland Barthes.

31   Lyrics from "In My Life", by Nelly, Avery Storm, Mase; songwriters Mason Betha, Ralph Distasio, Robert Gerongco, Cornell Haynes.

32   An entry from *Gravity's Rainbow*, by Thomas Pynchon.

33   An entry from *The Name of the Rose,* by Umberto Eco.

34   Lyrics from "Jim Jim Falls", by Morrissey.

35   Lyrics from "Help Me Make It Through the Night", by Elvis Presley.

36   The Old Norse word *gallin* is the root word of *gale force* and means "mad" or "insane."

37   Lyrics from "Help Me Make It Through the Night", by Elvis Presley.

38   *Being and Nothingness*, by Jean-Paul Sartre, weighed exactly one kilogram and was used by grocers in wartime Paris to replace the copper weights melted down for munitions.

39   Lyrics from "Run from Me", by Timber Timbre.

40   From Emily Dickinson's poem, "I measure every Grief I meet"; *The Poems of Emily Dickinson*, The Belnap Press of Harvard University Press.

41   Lyrics from "Milk It", by Kurt Cobain and Nirvana.

42   Count Ioannis Kapodistrias, the first governor of the Hellenic State, was on the 500 Greek Drachma note, taken out of circulation in 2002.

43   Lyrics from "I Contain Multitudes", by Bob Dylan.

44   COVID-19, or coronavirus, was a highly contagious, lethal pandemic that was first diagnosed in China in December 2019 and drove billions of people worldwide into quarantine.

45   "Hey Ya!", by Outkast, won 2004 Grammy Awards for Record of the Year, Best Urban/Alternative Performance and Best Music Video.

46   The entire country of Italy was ordered into quarantine on March 10, 2020.

47   *Salus Populi Romani* (*Protectress of the Roman People*), is thought to have been painted by Saint Luke, making it the first ever image depicting Madonna and Child.

48   Social distancing was a globally-recommended way to slow the spread of COVID-19.

49   From Canada.ca, the Government of Canada Website, on March 22, 2020.

50   The Prime Minister provided daily updates from Rideau Cottage during the pandemic. These instructions were offered on March 23, 2020.

51   From the Tuba Mirum, Requiem in B minor, Op. 89, Antonin Dvořák.

52   A headline from the March 20, 2020 edition of *The Globe and Mail*; article by Wency Leung.

53   Lyrics from "Jim Jim Falls", by Morrissey.

54   A headline in *Forbes* on March 24, 2020; article by Noma Nazish.

55   An entry from *Madness and Civilization*, by Michel Foucault.

56   Text from a video posted to the Pope's Twitter account on March 24, 2020.

57   The *Tao Te Ching* is a 6th-century Chinese text attributed to the philosopher Laozi, the founder of Taoism.

58   An entry from *Voyage Around My Room*, by Xavier de Maistre. De Maistre spent 42 days under house arrest in 1790 for duelling with a French military officer.

59   From "How can you feel safe amid coronavirus? Swap mindfulness for mindlessness", by Suzanne Moore; published in the March 30, 2020 edition of *The Guardian*.

60   By March 27, 2020, 11,591 people had died from COVID-19 in Italy.

61   From "Every day is now casual Friday, so embrace it", by Jen Zoratti; published in the April 1, 2020 edition of the *Winnipeg Free Press*.

62   As of April 3, 2020, more than a million people worldwide had been infected with coronavirus, with the death toll exceeding 52,000.

63   Lyrics from "Help Me Make It Through the Night", by Elvis Presley.

64   Wuhan, China, was wholly quarantined from the rest of the world for 76 days, beginning January 23, 2020.

65   COVID-19, and the resulting shutterings of economies around the world, created a global recession that, by early April 2020, was threatening to surpass the Great Depression in economic contraction.

66   The video-conferencing program Zoom surged in popularity during the COVID-19 pandemic.

67   Manitoba ordered all non-essential businesses closed on April 1, 2020.

68   From "The Ideas That Won't Survive the Coronavirus", by Viet Thanh Nguyen; published in the April 10, 2020 edition of *The New York Times*.

69   From "Will coronavirus signal the end of capitalism", by Paul Mason; published to web on April 3, 2020.

70   Rolling on the floor laughing.

71   An entry from *Death in Venice*, by Thomas Mann.

72   From "For those of us with depression, coronavirus is a double crisis", by Andrew Solomon; published in the April 13, 2020 edition of *The Guardian*.

73   An entry from *Madness and Civilization*, by Michel Foucault.

74   Lyrics from "I Contain Multitudes", by Bob Dylan.

75   An entry from *Gravity's Rainbow*, by Thomas Pynchon.

76   A reference to the main character in Umberto Eco's novel, *The Mysterious Flame of Queen Loana*.

77   An entry from *A Heart So White*, by Javier Marias.

78   Lyrics from "Blue Jeans", by Lana Del Rey.

79   An entry from *Dreamtigers*, by Jorge Luis Borges.

80   During the COVID-19 pandemic it was common, in many cities around the world, to applaud frontline care workers (such as doctors, nurses and paramedics) at a prescribed time in the early evenings.

81   Lyrics from "Spring Up O Well", by Phil Wickham.

82   From "In Praise of Pessimism: This country is going to need it Eeyores", by Jennifer Senior; published in the April 26, 2020 edition of *The New York Times*.

83   On April 23, 2020, United States President Donald Trump suggested the injection of disinfectants could combat COVID-19.

84   By the end of April 2020, the US economy had shrunk nearly 5% and economists were predicting an annual G.D.P

contraction of more than 30%. According to the UN, almost half the global workforce was in danger of losing their jobs.

85   An entry from *Mourning Diary*, by Roland Barthes.

86   An entry from Gerard Manley Hopkins' introduction to his volume, *Selected Poems*.

87   An entry from *Letters to a Young Poet*, by Rainer Maria Rilke.

88   Lyrics from "Help Me Make It Through the Night", by Elvis Presley.

89   References to *A Heart to White*, by Javier Marias.

90   Lyrics from "Where I End and You Begin", by Radiohead.

91   From Emily Dickinson's poem, "I measure every Grief I meet"; *The Poems of Emily Dickinson*, The Belnap Press of Harvard University Press.

92   A reference to a Javier Marias quote from his July 2006 interview with *The Independent*.

93   A reference to a line from *Time Regained,* by Marcel Proust.

Author Profile

Jerrad Peters lives in Winnipeg, Canada.

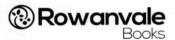

Publisher Information

Rowanvale Books provides publishing services to independent authors, writers and poets all over the globe. We deliver a personal, honest and efficient service that allows authors to see their work published, while remaining in control of the process and retaining their creativity. By making publishing services available to authors in a cost-effective and ethical way, we at Rowanvale Books hope to ensure that the local, national and international community benefits from a steady stream of good quality literature.

For more information about us, our authors or our publications, please get in touch.

www.rowanvalebooks.com
info@rowanvalebooks.com

CPSIA information can be obtained
at www.ICGtesting.com
Printed in the USA
LVHW101125150621
689924LV00035B/305/J